Color Atlas of
SMALL ANIMAL
DERMATOLOGY

Color Atlas of
SMALL ANIMAL DERMATOLOGY

BARBARA A. KUMMEL, D.V.M.

Animal Skin Disease Clinic
Rockville, Maryland

with **783** *four-color illustrations*

THE C. V. MOSBY COMPANY

ST. LOUIS • BALTIMORE • PHILADELPHIA • TORONTO   1990

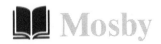

Editor: George Stamathis
Developmental editor: Elaine Steinborn
Project manager: Kathleen L. Teal
Book design: Liz Fett

Printed in the United States of America

The C.V. Mosby Company
11830 Westline Industrial Drive, St. Louis, Missouri 63146

Library of Congress Cataloging in Publication Data

Kummel, Barbara A.
    Color atlas of small animal dermatology / Barbara A. Kummel.
        p.   cm.
    Includes index.
    ISBN 0-8016-2910-1
    1. Dogs—Diseases—Atlases.   2. Cats—Diseases—Atlases.
3. Veterinary dermatology—Atlases.   I. Title.
    [DNLM: 1. Cat Diseases—atlases.   2. Dog Diseases—atlases.
3. Skin Diseases—veterinary—atlases.   SF 901 K96c]
SF992.S55K86   1989
636.089′65′0222—dc20
DNLM/DLC   89-9298
for Library of Congress   ˙CIP

C/W/W 9 8 7 6 5 4 3 2 1

PREFACE

The COLOR ATLAS OF SMALL ANIMAL DERMATOLOGY has been prepared as a guide to aid the general veterinary practitioner in recognizing and identifying various dermatologic diseases of the dog and cat. It is not meant to be a complete dermatology text and purposely lacks the pathogenesis of the various diseases, detailed disease descriptions, and current treatment modalities.

Many canine and feline skin diseases have similar clinical appearances. Therefore it is essential to develop a list of differential diagnoses from which to choose the correct diagnosis. An important aim of this atlas is to help the clinician compile this list of differential diagnoses. It has been organized to aid in this process. The final diagnosis can then be made based on signalment, careful history gathering, detailed physical examination, and appropriate diagnostic tests. Recognition of the disease is enhanced by the 783 color photographs in this book.

I would like to thank my father for encouraging my interest in and love of animals. In addition, my thanks to Dr. R. Gary Roop for initiating my interest in dermatology. Finally, thank you to my husband, Robert R. Banks, for his constant love and support.

Barbara A. Kummel

CONTENTS

COLOR ATLAS OF
SMALL ANIMAL
DERMATOLOGY

BACTERIAL DERMATOSES

Acute moist dermatitis (pyotraumatic dermatitis, hot spots)

Skin fold dermatitis

Superficial pustular dermatitis (puppy pyoderma, impetigo)

Bacterial folliculitis

Bacterial hypersensitivity-like dermatitis

Dermatophilosis

Bacterial furunculosis

German Shepherd Dog pyoderma

Nasal pyoderma

Chin pyoderma (canine acne)

Callous pyoderma

Bacterial cellulitis

Pododermatitis, (interdigital pyoderma, interdigital "cysts")

Atypical mycobacterial infection

Nocardiosis

Acute Moist Dermatitis (Pyotraumatic Dermatitis, Hot Spots)

CLINICAL SIGNS

1. Lesions produced by self-trauma such as licking, biting, and/or scratching
2. Typical lesions are circular or oval in shape, alopecic, erythematous, and moist or oozing
3. Surrounding skin and hair are usually normal
4. Intense pruritus

DIFFERENTIAL DIAGNOSIS

1. Demodicosis
2. Dermatophyte infection
3. Dermatophilosis
4. Neoplasia

UNDERLYING ETIOLOGIES

1. Flea bite hypersensitivity
2. Anal sacculitis
3. Irritating shampoos, insecticides, and chemicals
4. Intestinal parasite hypersensitivity
5. Allergic inhalant disease (atopy)
6. Poor grooming, especially matted hair
7. Otitis externa
8. Food hypersensitivity
9. Arthritis or other joint pain
10. Foreign bodies

DIAGNOSTIC AIDS

1. History of acute onset (usually a few hours)
2. Clinical appearance of lesion
3. Skin scrapings and fungal culture to rule out the two primary differential diagnoses
4. Skin biopsies for histopathologic examination usually not necessary

COMMENTS

Acute moist dermatitis is a common pruritic skin disorder of the dog. No age, breed, or sex predilection exists. Allergic patients are predisposed. Pathogenic bacteria are typically present on the surface of these lesions; however, the bacteria are simply colonizing and not invading the skin. Therefore antibiotic therapy is usually not necessary. However, "hot spots" on the faces of Golden Retrievers are frequently associated with a deep pyoderma and require antibiotic therapy. As with most skin diseases, successful treatment depends upon finding and treating the underlying etiology.

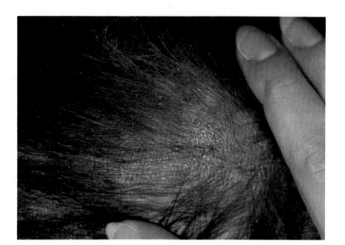

Figure 1-1 *Erythematous, moist lesion on hip of mixed-breed dog. Lesion was caused by pruritus resulting from flea bite hypersensitivity.*

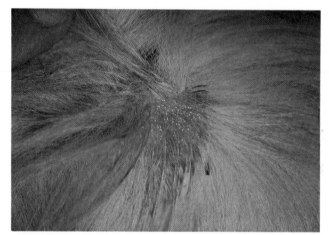

Figure 1-2 *Moist, weeping lesion on rump of 4-year-old Golden Retriever. Patient suffered from both flea bite hypersensitivity and allergic inhalant disease.*

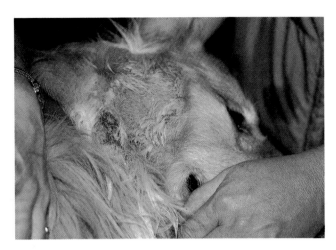

Figure 1-3 *Extensive "hot spot" on side of Golden Retriever's face. Patient's intense facial pruritus was secondary to allergic inhalant disease.*

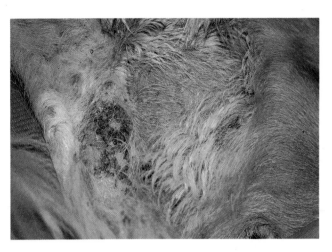

Figure 1-4 *Closer view of lesion shown in Figure 1-3.*

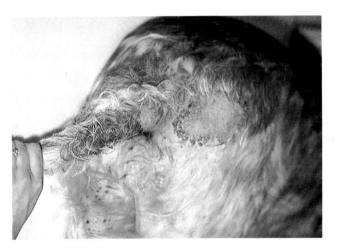

Figure 1-5 *Excoriated rump and tail of 7-year-old English Setter. Patient's severe self-trauma was initiated by flea bite hypersensitivity and anal sacculitis.*

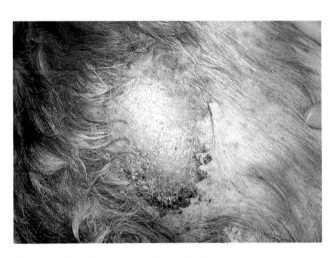

Figure 1-6 *Closer view of lesion in Figure 1-5.*

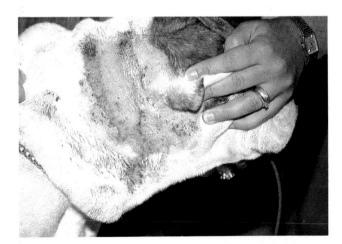

Figure 1-7 *Extensive "hot spot" on right side of English Bulldog's neck. Patient's pruritus resulted from otitis externa secondary to food hypersensitivity.*

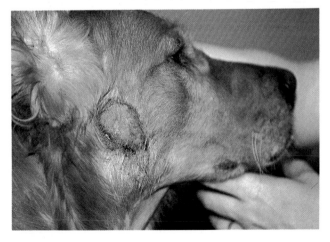

Figure 1-8 *This Golden Retriever's lesion was secondary to facial pruritus caused by allergic inhalant disease.*

Skin Fold Dermatitis

CLINICAL SIGNS

1. Lesions produced by friction and minor trauma usually associated with anatomical defects
2. Lesions are usually moist due to poor air circulation and trapped body secretions (sebum, saliva, tears, urine)
3. Secondary bacterial infection is common
4. Unpleasant odor often associated with lesions
5. Variable pruritus

TYPES OF SKIN FOLD DERMATITIS

1. Nasal fold
2. Facial fold
3. Tail fold
4. Lip fold
5. Body fold
6. Vulvar fold

DIAGNOSTIC AIDS

1. Location of lesion in any type of skin fold
2. Rule out demodicosis and dermatophyte infection

COMMENTS

Skin fold dermatitis is a common, chronic disorder in several breeds of dogs. No age or sex predilection exists. Predisposed breeds for facial and nasal fold dermatitis include English Bulldogs, Pugs, and Pekingese. Spaniels are more prone to develop lip fold dermatitis Tail fold dermatitis is common in dogs with corkscrew tails. Overweight patients have a tendency to develop body fold dermatitis. Skin fold dermatitis is rare in the cat.

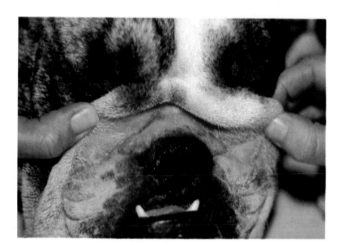

Figure 1-9 *Two-year-old English Bulldog with nasal fold dermatitis. Dermatitis was not evident until the fold was pulled back. Patient exhibited facial pruritus.*

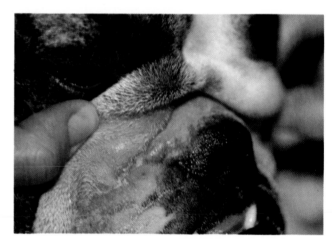

Figure 1-10 *Another view of lesion shown in Figure 1-9.*

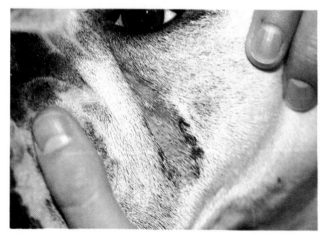

Figure 1-11 *English Bulldog with facial fold dermatitis. Patient's disease was unilateral and exacerbated by clogged tear duct.*

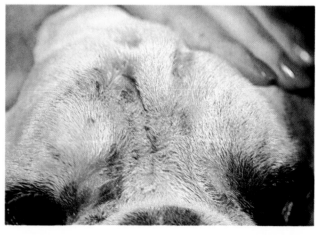

Figure 1-12 *"Forehead fold" dermatitis in excessively wrinkled English Bulldog.*

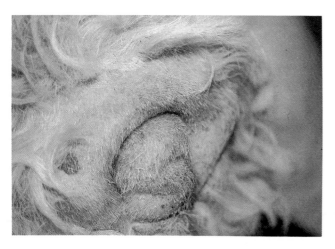

Figure 1-13 *West Highland White Terrier shows exuberant fat folds around tail base. Patient manifested rump pruritus.*

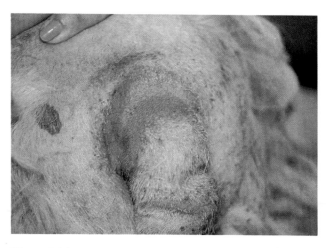

Figure 1-14 *Fat folds of patient shown in Figure 1-13 pulled cranially revealing weeping, erythematous lesions.*

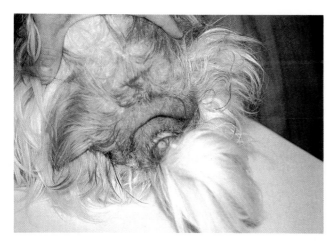

Figure 1-15 *Erythematous, exuberant tail base folds of a 9-year-old Shih Tzu. Patient suffered from chronic nonseasonal rump pruritus.*

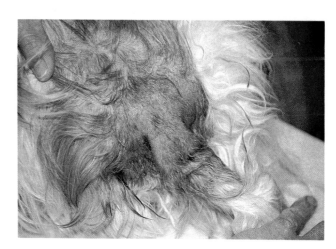

Figure 1-16 *Moist, erythematous lesions in tail fold area of patient shown in Figure 1-15. These lesions were only evident when skin folds were manually pulled forward.*

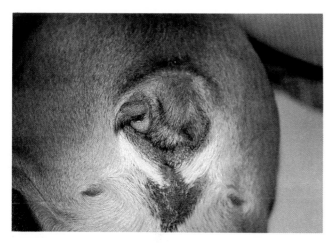

Figure 1-17 *Rear end of a "normal" Bulldog shows corkscrew tail.*

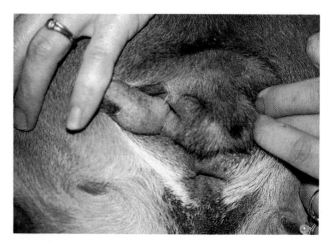

Figure 1-18 *Tail of patient shown in Figure 1-17 pulled laterally to reveal tail fold dermatitis that resulted in moderate degree of rear end pruritus.*

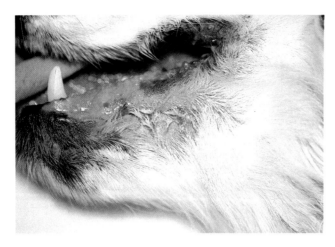

Figure 1-19 *Erythematous, foul-smelling, mildly pruritic dermatitis in lip fold of young English Springer Spaniel.*

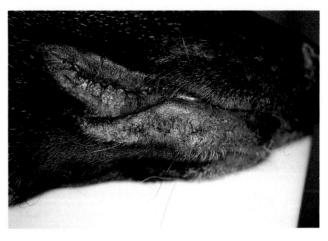

Figure 1-20 *Lip and lip fold lesions in a 6-year-old Labrador Retriever. Patient's lip dermatitis was secondary to chronic facial pruritus resulting from allergic inhalant disease.*

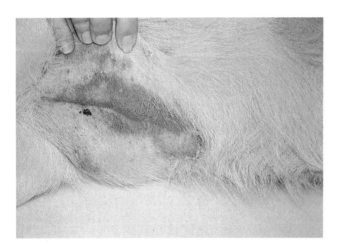

Figure 1-21 *Abdominal area of a 5-year-old overweight, mixed-breed dog. Skin fold is erythematous and moist. Secondary bacterial infection is evident.*

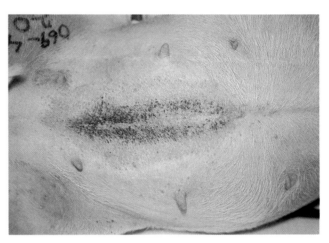

Figure 1-22 *Abdominal area of a 3-year-old Pit Bull Terrier shows body fold dermatitis. Involved area is erythematous with seborrheic exudate. (Part of tattoo is seen in upper left corner of photograph.)*

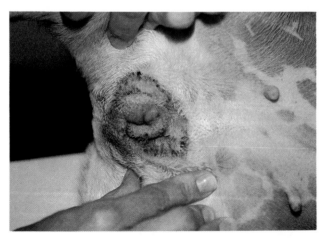

Figure 1-23 *Vulvar fold dermatitis in intact 4-year-old English Bulldog. Erythema and adherent seborrheic material are evident.*

Superficial Pustular Dermatitis (Puppy Pyoderma, Impetigo)

CLINICAL SIGNS

1. Small nonfollicular pustules
2. Ruptured pustules result in yellow crusts or scabs
3. Usually located in inguinal and/or axillary areas
4. Minimal to no pruritus

DIFFERENTIAL DIAGNOSIS

1. Demodicosis
2. Pemphigus foliaceus
3. Dermatophyte infection
4. Bacterial folliculitis

DIAGNOSTIC AIDS

1. Location of lesions
2. Age of patient (most patients are young)
3. Skin biopsies for histopathologic examination, usually not necessary but are diagnostic

COMMENTS

Superficial pustular dermatitis is most common in dogs under 6 months of age. There is no breed or sex predilection. In youngsters the disease may be associated with parasites, poor nutrition, or an unclean environment. Older dogs may develop the disease secondary to hypothyroidism, hyperadrenocorticism, or other debilitating diseases. Lesions in kittens are less common, usually located on the back and neck, and are associated with "mouthing" by their queens. The disease in dogs and cats is not contagious, as it is in humans.

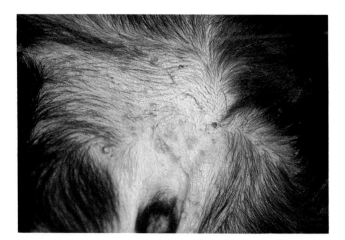

Figure 1-24   Nonfollicular pustules in inguinal area of 7-month-old male mixed Labrador Retriever.

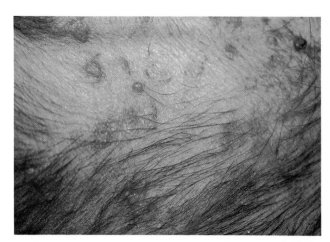

Figure 1-25   Closer view of pustules shown in Figure 1-24.

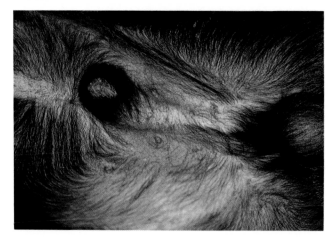

Figure 1-26   Pustules in groin of 10-month-old mixed-breed dog. Lesions were mildly pruritic and responded well to antibiotic therapy but recurred within a couple of weeks.

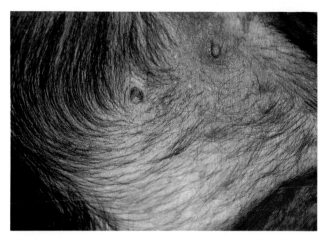

Figure 1-27   Closer view of nonfollicular pustules shown in Figure 1-26.

Bacterial Folliculitis

CLINICAL SIGNS

1. Small pustule with a hair shaft protruding from the center
2. Pustules are short-lived and may be difficult to find
3. Older lesions may appear as papules, crusts, and excoriations
4. In short-coated breeds hair in involved areas may stand on end, giving the coat a tufted appearance
5. Hair in involved areas may eventually be lost, giving the coat a moth-eaten appearance
6. Variable pruritus

DIFFERENTIAL DIAGNOSIS

1. Demodicosis
2. Dermatophyte infection
3. Urticaria
4. Superficial pustular dermatitis
5. Pemphigus foliaceus
6. Sarcoptic mange

UNDERLYING ETIOLOGIES

1. Flea bite hypersensitivity
2. Allergic inhalant disease (atopy)
3. Food hypersensitivity
4. Intestinal parasitism
5. Seborrheic dermatoses
6. Hypothyroidism

DIAGNOSTIC AIDS

1. Skin biopsies for histopathologic examination are diagnostic but rarely reveal underlying etiology
2. Skin scrapings and fungal culture to help rule out some differential diagnoses

COMMENTS

Bacterial folliculitis is a common presenting sign in canine skin disease. Short-coated breeds and younger animals may be predisposed. There is no sex predisposition. The degree of pruritus varies from marked to absent. Successful treatment of bacterial folliculitis, as is true with most dermatoses, depends upon detecting and treating the underlying etiology. Bacterial folliculitis is rare in the cat.

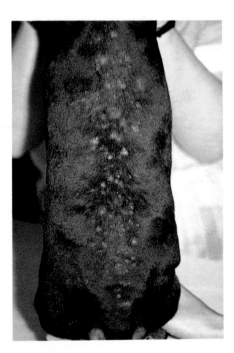

Figure 1-28 *Moth-eaten appearance to coat on back of 12-year-old Standard Shorthaired Dachshund. Patient's underlying disorder was hypothyroidism.*

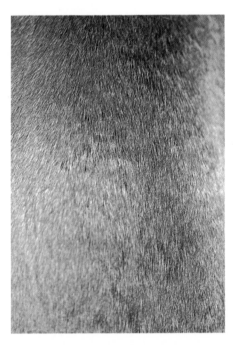

Figure 1-29 *Nonpruritic bacterial folliculitis on midback of young Great Dane. Patient's bacterial dermatitis may have been secondary to immature immune system.*

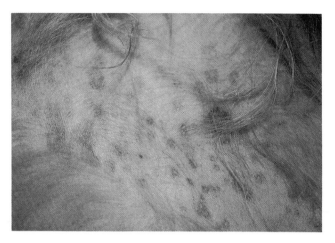

Figure 1-30 Papules and pustules on abdomen of Golden Retriever. Lesions were complication of allergic inhalant disease.

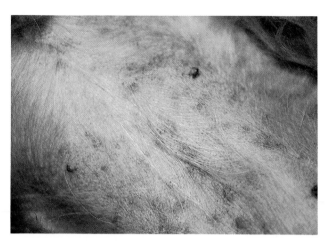

Figure 1-31 Folliculitis on abdomen of Cocker Spaniel. Lesions were secondary to flea bite hypersensitivity. (Part of tattoo is seen in upper right corner.)

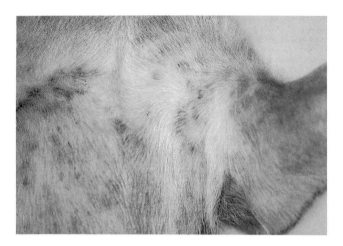

Figure 1-32 Axillary area of 5-year-old German Shepherd Dog. Patient's bacterial folliculitis was secondary to inflammation and pruritus caused by allergic inhalant disease (Atopy).

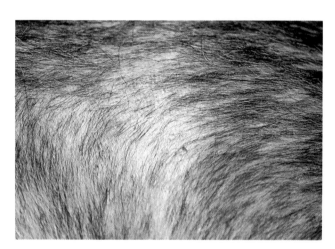

Figure 1-33 Bacterial lesions on lateral thoracic area of allergic patient shown in Figure 1-32.

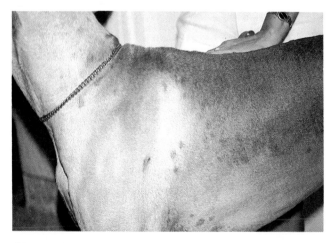

Figure 1-34 Left side of neck, chest, and thoracic areas of 3-year-old Great Dane. Areas of patient's coat that appear to be "moth eaten" are areas of bacterial folliculitis.

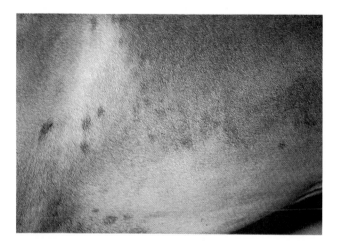

Figure 1-35 Closer view of bacterial lesions shown in Figure 1-34. Patient suffered from mild pruritus.

Bacterial Hypersensitivity-like Dermatitis

CLINICAL SIGNS

1. Circular erythematous lesions with raised, scaling peripheral borders
2. Older lesions may have central hyperpigmentation
3. Lesions may be located anywhere on the body; however, the head and legs are usually spared
4. Variable pruritus

DIFFERENTIAL DIAGNOSIS

1. True bacterial hypersensitivity dermatitis
2. Dermatophyte infection
3. Demodicosis
4. Lymphoreticular neoplasia

UNDERLYING ETIOLOGIES

1. Flea bite hypersensitivity
2. Allergic inhalant disease (atopy)
3. Food hypersensitivity
4. Endocrine imbalances
5. Seborrheic dermatoses

DIAGNOSTIC AIDS

1. Clinical appearance of the lesions
2. Skin biopsies for histopathologic examination

COMMENTS

Bacterial hypersensitivity-like dermatitis is a common presenting sign in many canine dermatologic disorders. No age or sex predilection exists. Long-haired dogs may be predisposed. The disease is not a true hypersensitivity reaction to staphylococcal bacteria. Rather, it is a bacterial dermatitis which is a cutaneous reaction to a myriad of underlying dermatologic disorders. Antibiotics are quite helpful, but unless the underlying etiology is detected and treated, the lesions recur. The disease has not been reported in the cat.

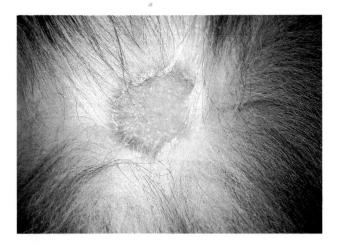

Figure 1-36 *Somewhat circular, erythematous lesion with scaling borders on lateral thorax of 10-year-old Collie. Underlying etiology of patient's bacterial dermatitis was diabetes mellitus.*

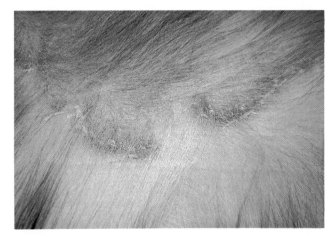

Figure 1-37 *More bacterial lesions on lateral thorax of patient shown in Figure 1-36.*

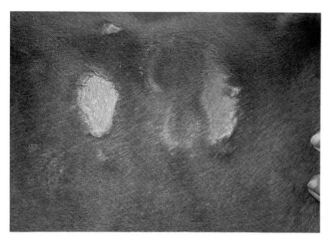

Figure 1-38 *Alopecic, mildly erythematous, scaling, nonpruritic lesions on lateral thorax of 8-year-old Dachshund with hypothyroidism.*

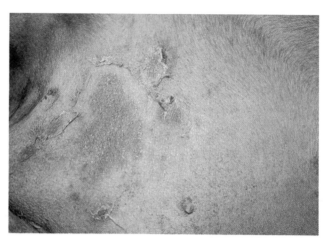

Figure 1-39 *More lesions on patient shown in Figure 1-38. Lesions responded temporarily to systemic antibiotics.*

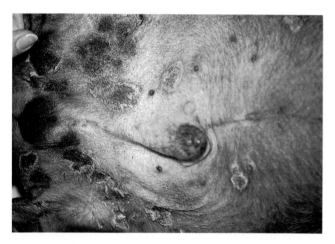

Figure 1-40 *Hyperpigmented, coalescing bacterial lesions on abdomen of 8-year-old Dachshund. Lesions were nonpruritic. Underlying etiology was hypothyroidism.*

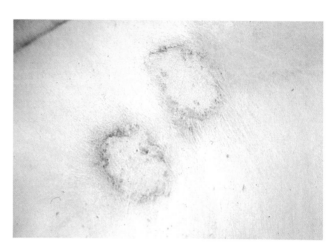

Figure 1-41 *Circular, alopecic, erythematous, scaling lesions in 5-year-old Samoyed.*

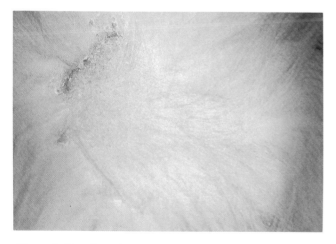

Figure 1-42 *Spreading bacterial lesion with erythematous, scaling border in 3-year-old dog with allergic inhalant disease (atopy).*

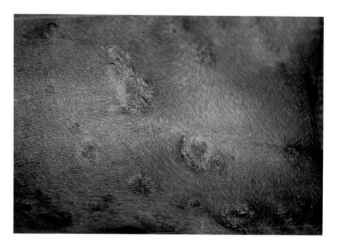

Figure 1-43 *Bacterial hypersensitivity-like lesions on chest of 11-year-old Dachshund with hyperadrenocorticism.*

Dermatophilosis

CLINICAL SIGNS

1. Exudative, purulent dermatitis covered by crusts
2. Seborrheic dermatitis
3. Chronic folliculitis
4. Moist surface dermatitis
5. Lesions are painful
6. Pruritus is mild to nonexistent

DIFFERENTIAL DIAGNOSIS

1. Surface pyodermas
2. Bacterial folliculitis
3. Demodicosis
4. Dermatophyte infection
5. Seborrheic dermatitis
6. Pemphigus foliaceus
7. Zinc dermatopathy

DIAGNOSTIC AIDS

1. Direct smear of the crusts and/or exudate stained with Diff Quick, Giemsa, Wright's, or Gram's reveal parallel rows of gram-positive cocci resembling "railroad tracks"
2. Skin biopsies for histopathologic examination are diagnostic

COMMENTS

Dermatophilosis is a rare disease which has been reported in dogs and cats. The causative organism is a gram-positive bacteria *Dermatophilus congolensis*. No age, breed, or sex predilection has been documented. Lesions are most commonly found on the dorsal back; however, any area of the body may be involved. *D. congolensis* is a secondary invader, so patients with excoriations, ectoparasites, matted and damp coats are predisposed.

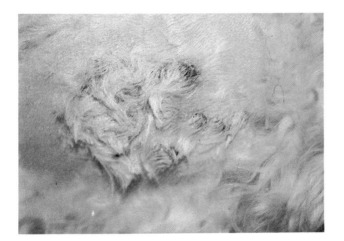

Figure 1-44 *Area of coalescing pustules, purulent exudate and matted hair on midback of mixed-breed dog. Lesion was painful and nonpruritic.*

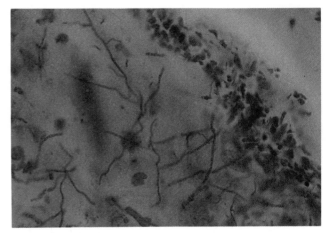

Figure 1-45 *Photomicrograph of skin biopsy from patient with dermatophilosis shows branching chains of cocci in epidermis.*

Bacterial Furunculosis

CLINICAL SIGNS

1. Deep pyoderma manifested by clusters of pustules, ulceration, and fistulization
2. Lesions typically discharge a hemopurulent exudate
3. Lesions may be generalized or localized
4. Pain and pruritus are variable

DIFFERENTIAL DIAGNOSIS

1. Atypical mycobacterial infection
2. Subcutaneous and systemic mycoses
3. Neoplasia

UNDERLYING ETIOLOGIES

1. Demodicosis
2. Hypothyroidism
3. Hyperadrenocorticism
4. Immune dysfunction
5. Immunosuppressive drugs
6. Foreign bodies

DIAGNOSTIC AIDS

1. Skin biopsies for histopathologic examination
2. Bacterial culture and sensitivity

COMMENTS

Bacterial furunculosis is a common presenting sign in many canine skin diseases. Youngsters and geriatric patients are predisposed. German Shepherd Dogs are predisposed (see German Shepherd Dog Pyoderma). No sex predilection exists. Bacterial furunculosis is almost always secondary to an underlying disease state. The disease is rare in the cat.

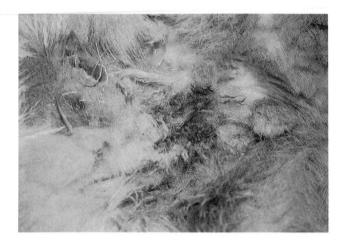

Figure 1-46 *Abdominal area of 8-year-old Malamute shows aggregations of pustules and ulceration. Patient's deep bacterial infection was secondary to high doses of corticosteroids prescribed to treat allergic dermatitis.*

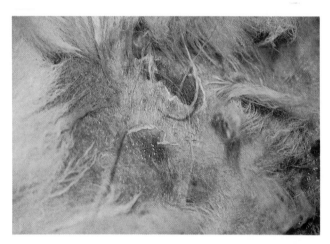

Figure 1-47 *Closer view of lesions shown in Figure 1-46.*

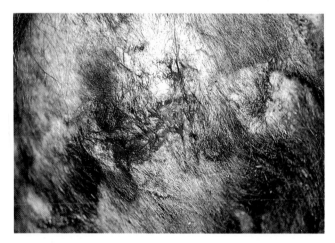

Figure 1-48 *Lateral thoracic area of mixed-breed dog shows coalescing ulcers and fistulous tracts.*

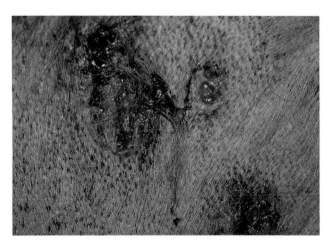

Figure 1-49 *Lateral thoracic area of 11-year-old mixed-breed dog. Note ulcerations and fistulous tracts surrounded by follicular plugging. Hyperadrenocorticism was underlying cause of dog's furunculosis.*

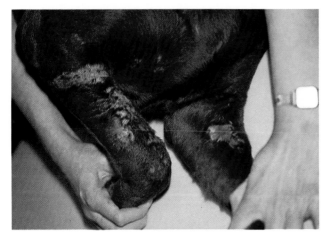

Figure 1-50 *Alopecia, inflammation, and ulceration on forelegs of chocolate Labrador Retriever. Patient's furunculosis was secondary to severe hypothyroidism.*

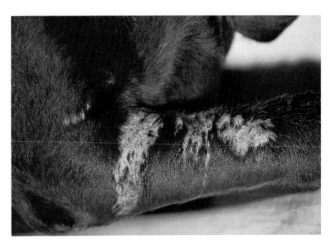

Figure 1-51 *Closer view of right foreleg of patient shown in Figure 1-50.*

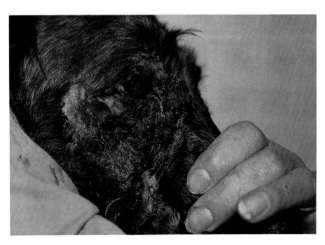

Figure 1-52 *Ulceration, fistulous tracts, and crusting on face of 7-year-old Scottish Terrier. Patient's recurrent bacterial furunculosis was related to flare-ups of allergic inhalant disease (Atopy).*

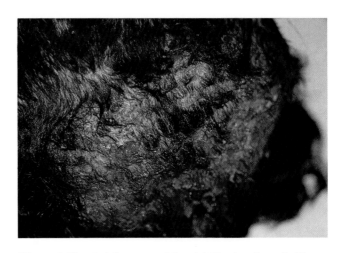

Figure 1-53 *Left hip area of Scottish Terrier shown in Figure 1-52. Again, note ulceration, fistulous tracts, and moist, purulent exudate.*

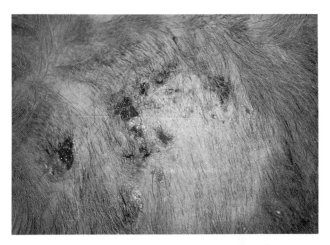

Figure 1-54 *Chest of 9-month-old Old English Sheepdog. Demodicosis was underlying etiology for patient's severe generalized bacterial furunculosis.*

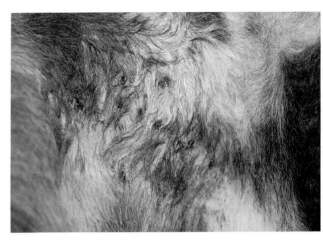

Figure 1-55 *Neck of patient shown in Figure 1-54. Note moist, matted hair and numerous ulcerations.*

German Shepherd Dog Pyoderma
CLINICAL SIGNS

1. Deep pyoderma manifested by clusters of pustules, ulceration, and fistulization
2. Any area of the body may be involved, but the rump and thoracic areas appear to be predisposed
3. Lesions typically exude a hemopurulent exudate
4. Pain and pruritus are variable

DIFFERENTIAL DIAGNOSIS

1. Demodicosis
2. Atypical mycobacterial infection
3. Subcutaneous and systemic mycoses
4. Neoplasia

DIAGNOSTIC AIDS

1. Skin biopsies for histopathologic examination
2. Bacterial culture and sensitivity

COMMENTS

German Shepherd Dog Pyoderma is a newly recognized canine skin disease. Middle-aged male dogs may be predisposed. Lesions are usually moderately pruritic and painful. Self-trauma such as licking and biting caused by an underlying allergic state (such as flea bite hypersensitivity and allergic inhalant disease) seems to initiate the pyoderma. There may also be an underlying immune deficiency disorder in these patients.

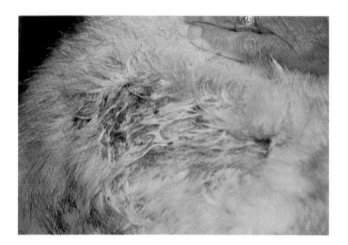

Figure 1-56 *Area of furunculosis on right hip of 6-year-old German Shepherd Dog. Note matted hair covering involved areas and hemopurulent exudate.*

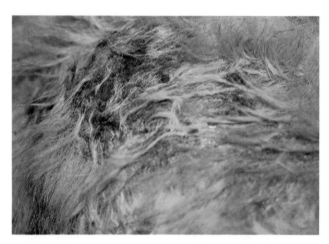

Figure 1-57 *Closer view of furunculosis shown in Figure 1-56.*

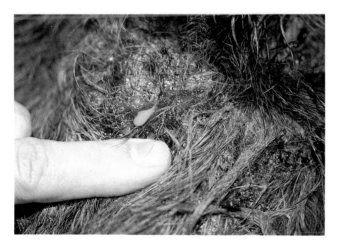

Figure 1-58 *Nine-year-old German Shepherd Dog shows purulent exudate from area of pyoderma on rump. Patient's disease was associated with hypothyroidism and flea bite hypersensitivity.*

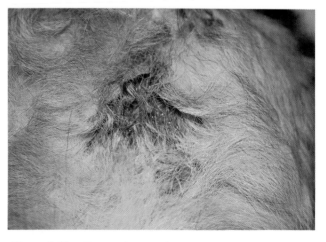

Figure 1-59 *Furunculosis on hip of German Shepherd Dog. Note matted, moist hair covering fistulous tracts.*

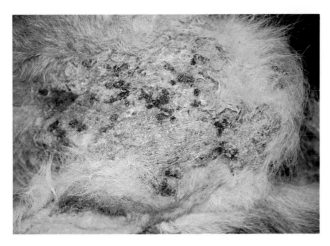

Figure 1-60 *Rump of 4-year-old German Shepherd Dog shows extensive area of furunculosis. Area is alopecic and hyperpigmented and has numerous fistulous tracts.*

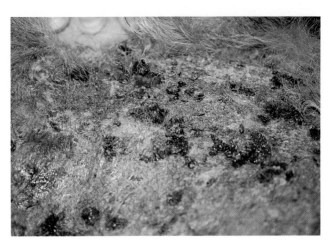

Figure 1-61 *Closer view of lesions shown in Figure 1-60. Lesions were mildly pruritic and somewhat painful.*

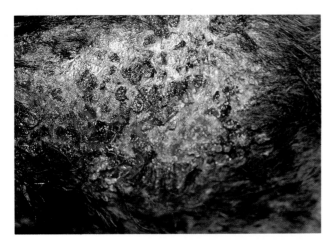

Figure 1-62 *Lateral thoracic area of German Shepherd Dog shows ulceration and crusting. Patient's furunculosis was exacerbated by allergic inhalant disease (atopy).*

Nasal Pyoderma

CLINICAL SIGNS

1. Folliculitis and furunculosis on bridge of the nose
2. Area is usually quite swollen and painful
3. Surface ulceration is common
4. Other areas of the body are usually not involved

DIFFERENTIAL DIAGNOSIS

1. Demodicosis
2. Pemphigus erythematosus, foliaceus, or vulgaris
3. Systemic or discoid lupus erythematosus
4. Nasal solar dermatitis
5. Superficial or deep mycotic infection
6. Zinc dermatopathy
7. Neoplastic disease
8. Juvenile pyoderma (puppy strangles)
9. Drug eruption

DIAGNOSTIC AIDS

1. Biopsies for histopathologic examination
2. Clinical appearance and location of lesions

COMMENTS

Nasal pyoderma is an uncommon disease of the dog. It has not been reported in the cat. No age or sex predilections exist. Long-nosed (dolichocephalic) breeds of dogs such as German Shepherd Dogs and Collies are predisposed. The etiology is unknown, but lesions may start with self-induced trauma such as rooting and digging. Pustules are the early lesions; however, furunculosis soon develops. Disease progression is quite rapid. Scarring may result.

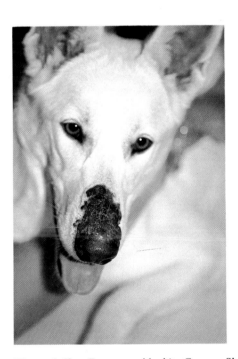

Figure 1-63 Two-year-old white German Shepherd Dog has extensive swelling, ulceration, and crusting of bridge of nose. Area was quite painful and nonpruritic.

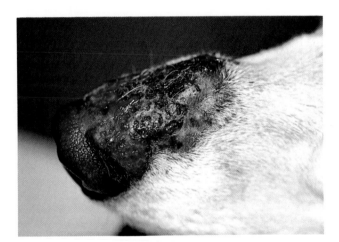

Figure 1-64 Close-up photograph of patient's nose shown in Figure 1-63. The degree of swelling and ulceration is quite evident.

Chin Pyoderma (Canine Acne)

CLINICAL SIGNS

1. Lesions in mild cases consist of papules and pustules with minimal erythema and swelling. Discomfort is usually not associated with mild cases.
2. Lesions in more severe cases consist of furuncles with marked swelling and erythema. These lesions often exude a hemopurulent exudate and may be quite painful.

DIFFERENTIAL DIAGNOSIS

1. Demodicosis
2. Juvenile pyoderma (puppy strangles)
3. Foreign body

DIAGNOSTIC AIDS

1. Location and appearance of the lesions
2. Skin scrapings to rule out demodicosis
3. Biopsies for histopathologic examination are helpful but may not be necessary

COMMENTS

Chin pyoderma is most common in short-coated breeds of dogs. It usually starts at less than 1 year of age. Mild cases often persist for 2 to 3 months and may be self-limiting. More severe cases require systemic antibiotics as well as topical treatment. In persistent cases the possible underlying etiologies of hypothyroidism and immune deficiency states should be investigated.

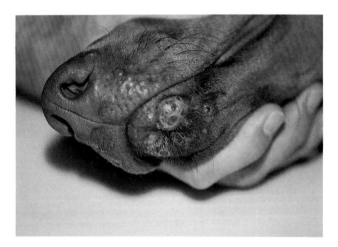

Figure 1-65   *Ulcerated furuncle surrounded by pustules on chin of 9-month-old Doberman Pinscher.*

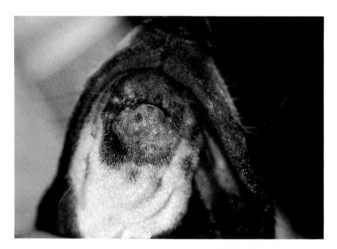

Figure 1-66   *Pustules and furuncles on chin of 7-month-old mixed Beagle. Lesions were nonpainful and nonpruritic.*

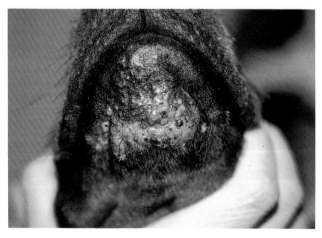

Figure 1-67   *Coalescing papules and pustules with some exudation on chin of 2-year-old mixed-breed dog. Alopecia and hyperpigmentation of lips are result of chronic inflammation.*

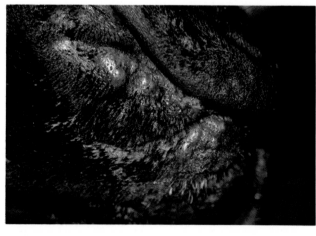

Figure 1-68   *Numerous pustules on lips and chin of young English Mastiff.*

Callous Pyoderma

CLINICAL SIGNS

1. Deep pyoderma manifested by clusters of pustules, ulceration, and fistulization
2. Lesions may discharge a hemopurulent exudate
3. Lesions usually involve the elbows, hocks, and/or sternum.

DIFFERENTIAL DIAGNOSIS

1. Foreign body
2. Neoplasia
3. Demodicosis

DIAGNOSTIC AIDS

1. Clinical appearance and location of lesion
2. Biopsies for histopathologic examination are helpful but usually not necessary)

COMMENTS

Callous pyoderma usually affects larger breeds of dogs. Great Danes, Doberman Pinschers, and Saint Bernards may be predisposed to elbow pyoderma. Sternal callous pyoderma is more common in Dachshunds and Irish Setters. (Refer to "Callouses" in Section 8.) No age or sex predilections exist. Overweight patients and hypothyroid patients are predisposed.

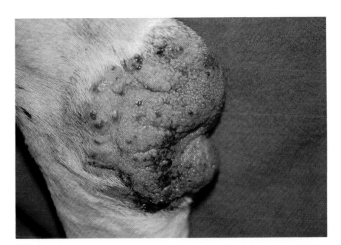

Figure 1-69 Numerous pustules on swollen elbow of Great Dane. Hypothyroidism was contributing factor in patient's pyoderma.

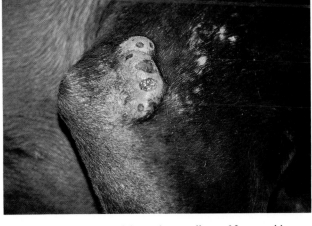

Figure 1-70 Ulcerated furuncles on elbow of 2-year-old Doberman Pinscher.

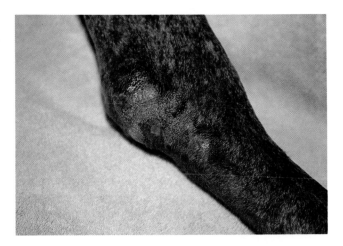

Figure 1-71 Pyoderma on Bull Mastiffs' calloused hock.

Bacterial Cellulitis

CLINICAL SIGNS

1. Deep suppurative bacterial infection
2. Areas of infection poorly defined
3. Erythema, swelling, and pain are common features
4. Pruritus is minimal to absent

DIFFERENTIAL DIAGNOSIS

1. Furunculosis
2. Demodicosis
3. Nonseptic edema
4. Neoplastic disease
5. Atypical mycobacterial infections
6. Juvenile pyoderma (puppy strangles)

DIAGNOSTIC AIDS

1. Skin biopsies for histopathologic examination
2. Bacterial culture and sensitivity of skin biopsies

COMMENTS

Bacterial cellulitis is an uncommon sequela to deep bacterial infections in dogs. The infection dissects through tissue planes. No age, breed, or sex predispositions exist. In cats the disease often results from fight wounds. Edema and pain are common features. Patients are usually febrile, lethargic, and anorectic. Involved areas may slough, giving rise to large ulcerated areas that frequently heal by scar tissue formation.

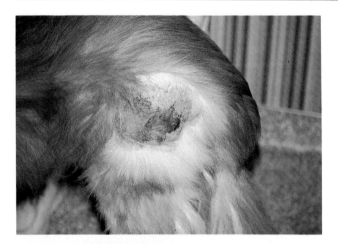

Figure 1-72   Marked swelling with erythema and surface pyoderma on left hip of Golden Retriever. Patient's cellulitis was secondary to a dog fight wound.

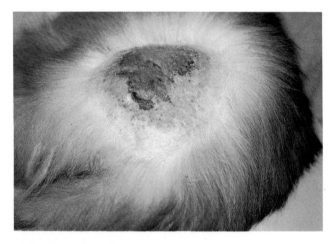

Figure 1-73   Closer view of lesion shown in Figure 1-72.

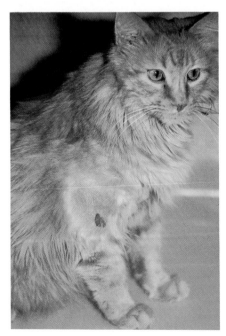

Figure 1-74   Three-year-old cat shows area of erythema and swelling secondary to a puncture wound. Lesion was painful and mildly pruritic.

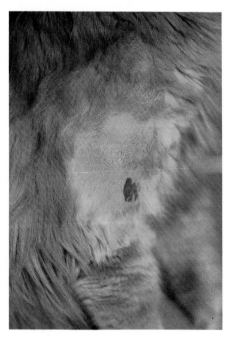

Figure 1-75   Closer view of lesion shown in Figure 1-74.

Pododermatitis **21**

Pododermatitis
(Interdigital Pyoderma)
(Interdigital "Cysts")

CLINICAL SIGNS

1. Fistulas, ulcers, and/or nodules may be present
2. Skin in affected interdigital spaces is erythematous and edematous
3. The lesions are *not* cysts, as they often are mistakenly described
4. A serosanguinous or purulent exudate may be observed

UNDERLYING ETIOLOGIES

1. Demodicosis
2. Bacterial infection
3. Dermatophyte infection
4. Allergic inhalant disease
5. Local injury
6. Contact with irritants
7. Sterile pyogranulomas
8. Intestinal parasitism
9. Hypothyroidism
10. Foreign body
11. Neoplasia

DIAGNOSTIC AIDS

1. Skin scrapings to rule out demodicosis
2. Bacterial and fungal cultures, may be indicated
3. Skin biopsies for histopathologic examination may be helpful, but they rarely detect the underlying etiology

COMMENTS

Pododermatitis is a common dermatologic disorder of the dog. It is much less common in the cat. No age or sex predilection exists. Short-coated breeds of dogs appear to be predisposed. Determining the underlying etiology is essential for successful treatment.

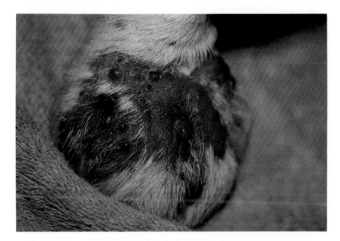

Figure 1-76 Swollen forefoot of Beagle with demodicosis. Note erythema, swelling, and numerous hemorrhagic pustules.

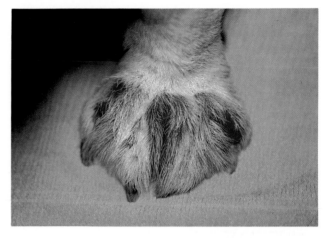

Figure 1-77 Interdigital erythema and pustules on forefoot of 5-year-old mixed-breed dog.

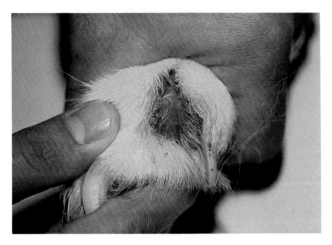

Figure 1-78 *Interdigital erythema, exudation, and bacterial dermatitis in Siberian Husky with allergic inhalant disease.*

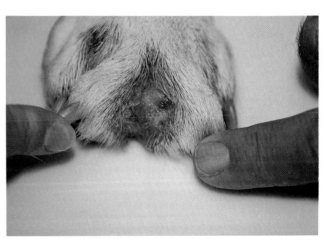

Figure 1-79 *Forefoot of 5-year-old yellow Labrador Retriever with hypothyroidism. Note marked interdigital erythema with fistulous tracts and exudate.*

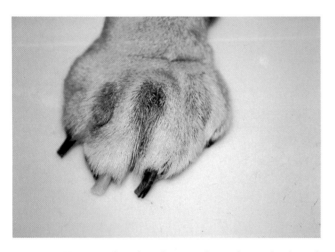

Figure 1-80 *Interdigital erythema and pustules on forefoot of 5-year-old mixed-breed dog. Etiology of patient's bacterial pododermatitis was not detected.*

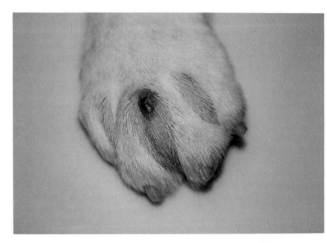

Figure 1-81 *Hemorrhagic pustule and interdigital erythema on forefoot of English Bulldog. Factors contributing to patient's pododermatitis included allergic inhalant disease (atopy), obesity, and hypothyroidism.*

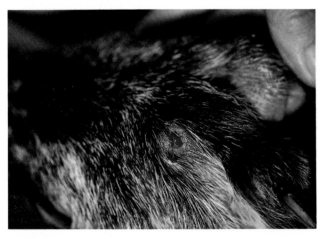

Figure 1-82 *Interdigital pustule on forefoot of German Shorthaired Pointer. Patient's pododermatitis was probably foreign body induced.*

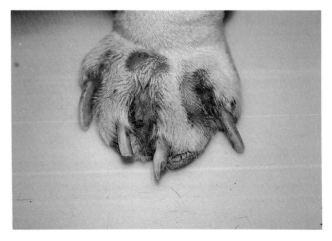

Figure 1-83 *Swelling, interdigital erythema, and exudation on forefoot of English Bulldog. Underlying etiology was demodicosis.*

Atypical Mycobacterial Infection

CLINICAL SIGNS

1. Ulcers, draining tracts, and fistulas
2. Lesions typically appear as a "nonhealing wound"
3. A clear, or cloudy, slimey exudate is present
4. Lesions develop slowly over a period of several weeks or several months
5. Abdominal area, inguinal, and rump are the most common sites of involvement
6. Patients are mildly to nonpruritic
7. Pain may be associated with lesions
8. Signs of systemic illness may be present

DIFFERENTIAL DIAGNOSIS

1. Feline leprosy
2. Cutaneous tuberculosis
3. Nocardiosis
4. Deep mycotic infections
5. Bacterial furunculosis
6. Demodicosis
7. Neoplasia

DIAGNOSTIC AIDS

1. Acid-fast organisms are rarely found on direct smears of the exudate
2. Cultures of the exudate and excised tissue may grow the organism. Blood agar, Löwenstein-Jensen, or Stonebrink's medium should be used
3. Skin biopsies for histopathologic examination may be helpful

COMMENTS

Atypical mycobacterial infection is more common in the cat than in the dog. No age, breed, or sex predilections have been recognized. Lesions are initiated by an injury such as a fight or puncture wound which develops into a subcutaneous abscess and draining tract. The causative organisms include the following Mycobacterium; *fortuitum, chelonei, smegmatis, phlei,* and *xenopi.* The infection responds poorly to treatment.

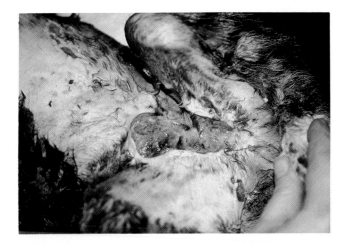

Figure 1-84 *Abdominal and inguinal areas of young Domestic Short-Haired cat shows extensive ulceration caused by* Mycobacterium fortuitum.

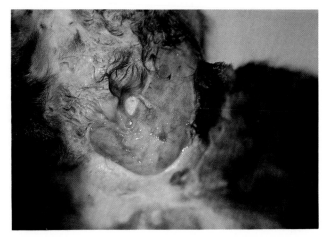

Figure 1-85 *Abdomen of 7-year-old mixed-breed cat shows 8×3 cm ulceration. Lesion occurred after ovariohysterectomy. Causative organism was* Mycobacterium smegmatis.

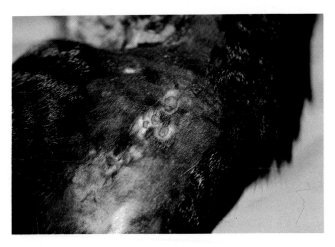

Figure 1-86 *Rump of Domestic Short-Haired cat shows circular ulcerations. Lesions were caused by* Mycobacterium fortuitum *and were most likely initiated by puncture wound from cat fight.*

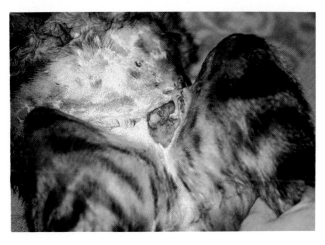

Figure 1-87 *Ulcerated abdominal area of 2-year-old cat caused by* Mycobacterium fortuitum.

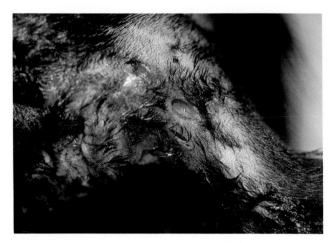

Figure 1-88 *Tail and tail base of 11-year-old cat with* Mycobacterium smegmatis *infection. Infection was initiated by cat fight wound.*

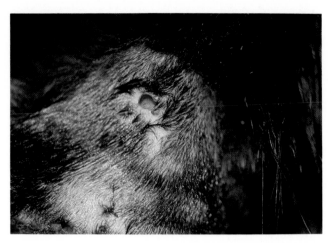

Figure 1-89 *Another atypical mycobacterial lesion from patient shown in Figure 1-88.*

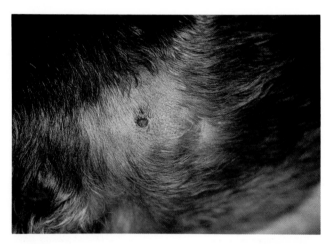

Figure 1-90 *Ulcerated lesion caused by* Mycobacterium smegmatis *in Lhasa Apso.*

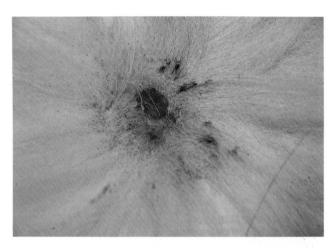

Figure 1-91 *Thirteen-year-old Shetland Sheepdog with* Mycobacterium fortuitum *infection. Patient's disease involved entire trunk.*

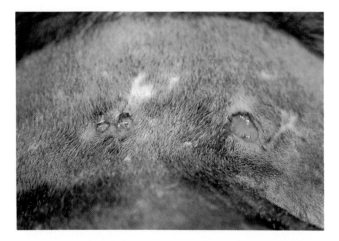

Figure 1-92 *Shaved lateral thoracic area of mixed-breed dog. Atypical mycobacterial ulcerations are somewhat circular and have moist, slimey surface.*

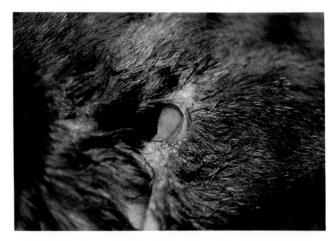

Figure 1-93 *Flank area of Calico cat. This* Mycobacterium smegmatis *lesion is circular and exuding serous material.*

Nocardiosis

CLINICAL SIGNS

1. First clinical sign is often a cutaneous injury that does not respond to treatment
2. Fistulous tracts draining a "tomato soup" exudate
3. Abscesses, ulcerated nodules, and cellulitis
4. A pulmonary form of the disease also exists

DIFFERENTIAL DIAGNOSIS

1. Tuberculosis
2. Atypical mycobacterial infection
3. Deep mycotic infections
4. Chronic bacterial infection
5. Neoplasia

DIAGNOSTIC AIDS

1. Biopsies for histopathologic examination may reveal nodular-to-diffuse panniculitis or dermatitis or both. Tissue grains may or may not be present
2. A Gram stain of the exudate reveals gram-positive, branching, beaded filaments
3. Culture of the exudate on blood agar and plain Sabouraud dextrose agar plates may be diagnostic

COMMENTS

Nocardiosis is an uncommon disease of the dog. It is caused most frequently by the organisms *Nocardia asteroides* and *N. brasiliensis*. The organisms are aerobic, gram-positive, have branching filaments, and are partially acid-fast. *N. asteroides* is a common soil saprophyte and is worldwide in distribution. The organisms may be inhaled or ingested but often enter the body through a cutaneous injury site.

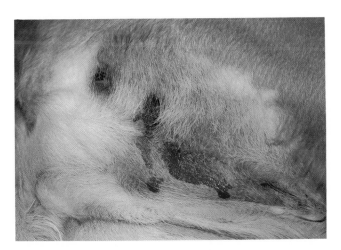

Figure 1-94 *Draining lesions on caudal thigh of 3-year-old mixed-breed dog. Biopsies of lesions revealed nodular panniculitis. The organism,* Nocardia asteroides *was found on culture of exudate.*

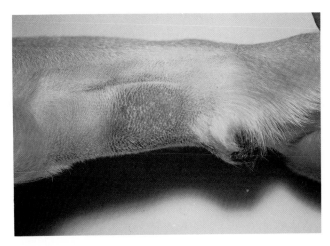

Figure 1-95 *Soft, painful nodule on foreleg of Golden Retriever. Culture of tissue section of lesion revealed* Nocardia asteroides.

HYPERSENSITIVITY (ALLERGIC) DERMATOSES

Canine allergic inhalant disease (atopy)

Feline allergic inhalant disease (atopy)

Canine flea bite hypersensitivity

Feline flea bite hypersensitivity

Canine food hypersensitivity

Feline food hypersensitivity

Allergic contact dermatitis

Flea collar contact dermatitis

Intestinal parasite hypersensitivity

Hormonal hypersensitivity

Urticaria and angioedema (hives)

Drug eruption

True bacterial hypersensitivity (staphylococcal hypersensitivity)

Canine Allergic Inhalant Disease (Atopy)

CLINICAL SIGNS

1. Pruritus typically involving the face, feet, and ventrum; however, any and all areas of the body may be pruritic
2. Alopecia, erythema, hyperpigmentation, and lichenification are common secondary sequelae to pruritus
3. Otitis externa
4. Conjunctivitis
5. Anal sacculitis
6. Secondary bacterial dermatitis
7. Secondary seborrheic dermatoses
8. Acral lick dermatitis (lick granulomas)
9. Less than 5% of patients show upper respiratory signs such as sneezing and coughing

DIFFERENTIAL DIAGNOSIS

1. Flea bite hypersensitivity
2. Food hypersensitivity
3. Intestinal parasite hypersensitivity
4. Contact dermatitis
5. Sarcoptic mange
6. Demodicosis
7. True bacterial hypersensitivity

DIAGNOSTIC AIDS

1. A thoroughly taken history is the most important diagnostic aid
2. Complete intradermal skin testing
3. Preliminary studies show that Radio-Allergo-Sorbent (RAST) and Enzyme-Linked Immuno-Sorbent Assay (ELISA) in vitro testing may be less accurate than complete intradermal skin testing
4. Skin biopsies for histopathologic examination may rule out differential diagnoses but they are not diagnostic for inhalant allergies

COMMENTS

Canine allergic inhalant disease is a common cause of pruritic skin disease and otitis in the dog. Clinical signs most frequently begin between 4 months and 4 years of age. Disease incidence is slightly higher in females. The disease is genetically programmed with many breeds being predisposed. However, allergic inhalant disease has been recognized in virtually every breed.

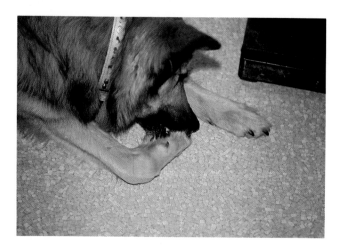

Figure 2-1   *Patient with allergic inhalant disease demonstrates pedal pruritus, which is one of most common signs.*

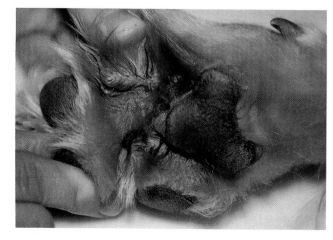

Figure 2-2   *Interdigital area of forefoot of patient in Figure 2-1 shows self-induced inflammation.*

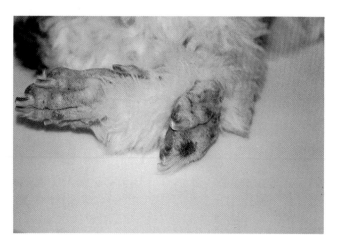

Figure 2-3   *Self-induced alopecia and erythema on forefeet of Old English Sheepdog with allergic inhalant disease.*

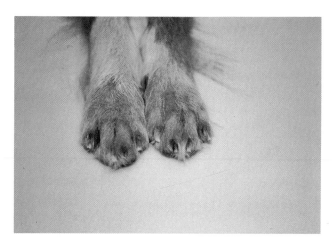

Figure 2-4   *Forefeet of 5-year-old Shetland Sheepdog with allergic inhalant disease show self-induced alopecia and erythema.*

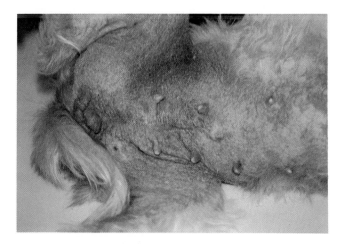

Figure 2-5   *Abdominal area of allergic mixed-breed dog shows hyperpigmentation and lichenification secondary to chronic licking.*

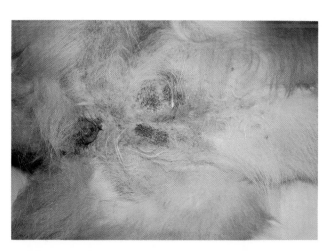

Figure 2-6   *Self-induced alopecia, erythema, and bacterial dermatitis of abdominal area of allergic Golden Retriever.*

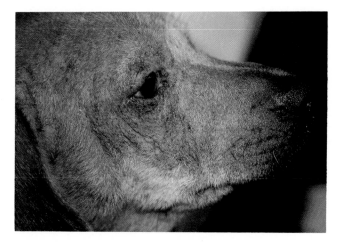

Figure 2-7   *Self-induced alopecia, erythema, hyperpigmentation, and lichenification on face of allergic patient.*

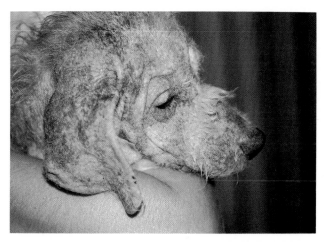

Figure 2-8   *Severe alopecia, erythema, lichenification, and crusts on face of 7-year-old dog with chronic allergies.*

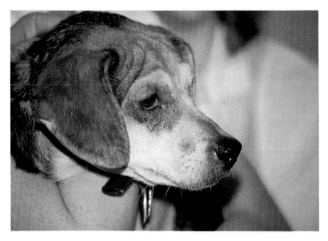

Figure 2-9 *Four-year-old allergic Beagle with allergic inhalant disease has self-induced periocular alopecia with erythema and hyperpigmentation.*

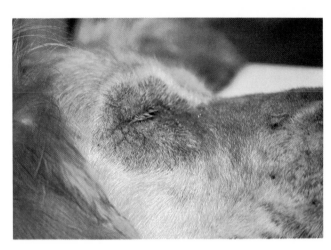

Figure 2-10 *Golden Retriever with periocular irritation caused by facial pruritus.*

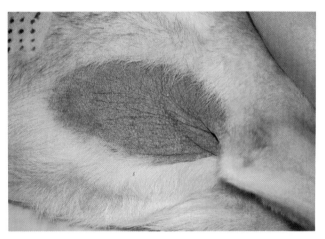

Figure 2-11 *Axillary area of German Shepherd Dog. Alopecia and hyperpigmentation are secondary to chronic pruritus. (Edge of intradermal skin test is evident in upper left corner.)*

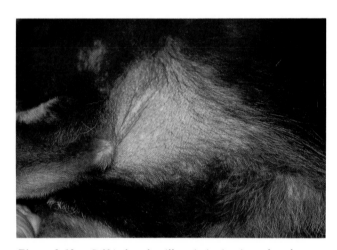

Figure 2-12 *Self-induced axillary irritation in a chocolate Labrador Retriever.*

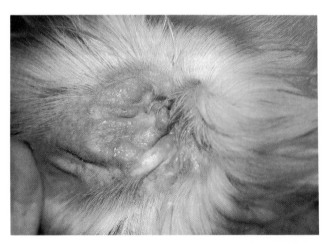

Figure 2-13 *Otitis externa in Golden Retriever with inhalant allergies. Most cases of allergic otitis are bilateral; however, occasionally the otitis is unilateral.*

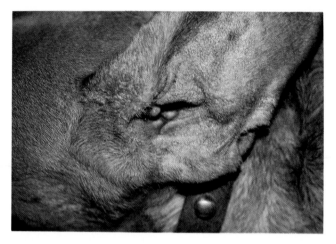

Figure 2-14 *Seborrheic otitis externa in Dachshund with allergic inhalant disease. Otitis may be the only clinical sign in allergic patient.*

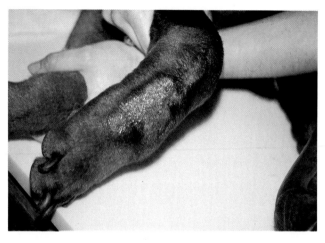

Figure 2-15 *Acral lick dermatitis on foreleg of Doberman Pinscher with inhalant allergies. Lesions are created by chronic licking and chewing of area.*

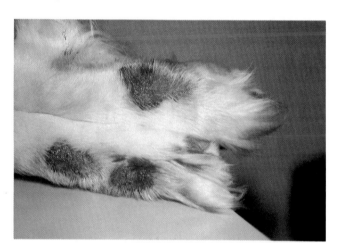

Figure 2-16 *Mixed-breed allergic patient with acral lick dermatitis on forelegs. These self-induced lesions are most commonly found on forelegs; however, all four legs may be involved.*

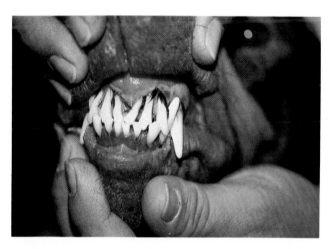

Figure 2-17 *Three-year-old Doberman Pinscher with inhalant allergies. Chronic chewing and licking resulted in erosion of gums and lodging of hair between teeth and gums.*

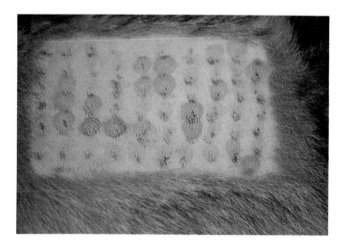

Figure 2-18 *Intradermal skin test using 61 injections (four controls and 57 antigens). This patient's positive reactions are quite evident.*

Feline Allergic Inhalant Disease (Atopy)

CLINICAL SIGNS

1. Head and neck pruritus
2. Self-induced alopecia
3. Eosinophilic plaque lesions
4. Miliary dermatitis

DIFFERENTIAL DIAGNOSIS

1. Flea bite hypersensitivity
2. Food hypersensitivity
3. Dermatophyte infection
4. Notoedric mange
5. Cheyletiella dermatitis
6. *Otodectes cynotis* (ear mites)
7. Intestinal parasite hypersensitivity
8. Contact dermatitis
9. Psychogenic alopecia
10. Feline "endocrine" alopecia

DIAGNOSTIC AIDS

1. Thorough history
2. Multiple skin scrapings, allergy test diet, and fecal floatations to help rule out other differential diagnoses
3. Complete intradermal skin testing
4. Skin biopsies for histopathologic examination may help rule out other differential diagnoses; however, they are not diagnostic for inhalant allergies

COMMENTS

Allergic inhalant disease is a newly recognized cause of pruritus, miliary dermatitis, and eosinophilic plaques in the cat. Signs usually begin between 1 and 6 years of age. No breed or sex predilection has been recognized. The bilaterally symmetric self-induced alopecia seen in felines with inhalant allergies may have been previously misdiagnosed as psychogenic alopecia and/or feline endocrine alopecia.

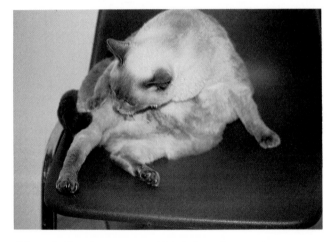

Figure 2-19 *Siamese cat with inhalant allergies demonstrates abdominal and inguinal area pruritus.*

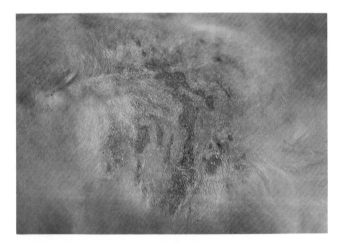

Figure 2-20 *Self-induced abdominal area lesions of patient shown in Figure 2-19.*

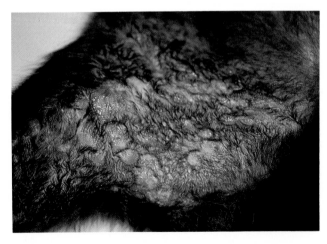

Figure 2-21 *Self-induced eosinophilic plaques on medial aspect of rear leg of 5-year-old cat with inhalant allergies.*

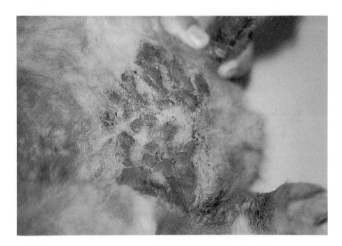

Figure 2-22 *Abdominal area of cat with pollen allergies shows numerous eosinophilic plaques.*

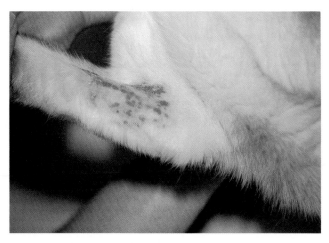

Figure 2-23   *Medial aspect of right foreleg of 7-year-old cat with inhalant allergies. Biopsies of self-induced lesions revealed eosinophilic plaques.*

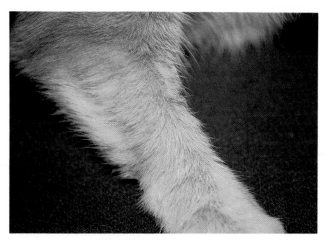

Figure 2-24   *Self-induced alopecia and erythema of right foreleg of Domestic Short-Haired cat with dust and mold allergies.*

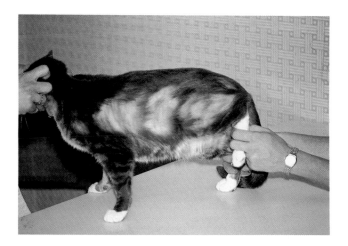

Figure 2-25   *Inhalant allergic 3-year-old cat with bilaterally symmetric, self-induced truncal alopecia.*

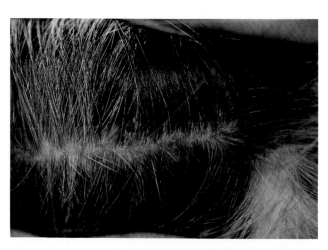

Figure 2-26   *Miliary dermatitis on midback of long-haired cat with inhalant allergies. Lesions are also commonly seen in felines with flea bite and food hypersensitivities.*

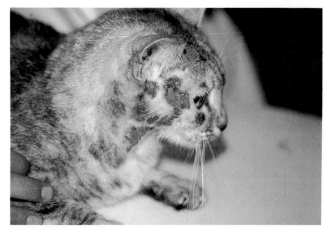

Figure 2-27   *Severe head and neck excoriations in Domestic Short-Haired cat. Head and neck pruritus is common sign of feline inhalant allergy.*

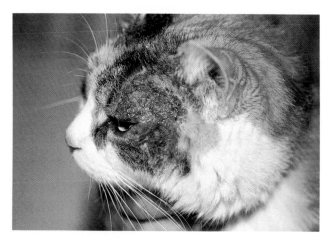

Figure 2-28   *Inhalant allergic Calico cat with preauricular excoriations.*

Canine Flea Bite Hypersensitivity

CLINICAL SIGNS

1. Pruritus mainly involving rump, tail, rear legs, and inguinal area
2. In some cases the pruritus is generalized
3. Self-induced alopecia
4. Secondary hyperpigmentation and lichenification
5. Acute moist dermatitis (hot spots)
6. Secondary bacterial dermatitis
7. Secondary seborrheic dermatoses
8. Otitis externa

DIFFERENTIAL DIAGNOSIS

1. Allergic inhalant disease (atopy)
2. Food hypersensitivity
3. Intestinal parasite hypersensitivity
4. Other causes of bacterial dermatitis
5. Other causes of seborrheic dermatoses
6. Sarcoptic mange

DIAGNOSTIC AIDS

1. Finding fleas and/or flea excreta on patient with "classic" clinical signs (always use flea comb)
2. Positive reaction to intradermally injected flea antigen
3. Response to flea eradication program

COMMENTS

Flea bite hypersensitivity is the most common cause of allergic dermatitis in the dog. No breed or sex predilections have been documented. The average age at onset is 2 to 7 years. Patients with allergic inhalant disease may be predisposed. Flea bite hypersensitivity most likely involves both immediate and delayed-type hypersensitivity reactions.

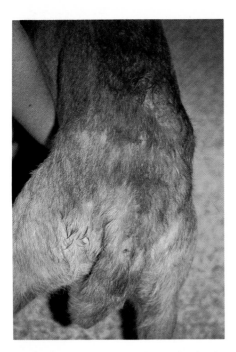

Figure 2-29   *Rump of yellow Labrador Retriever shows numerous areas of self-induced acute moist dermatitis or "hot spots".*

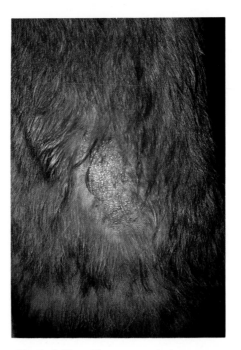

Figure 2-30   *Closer view of "hot spot" on flea allergic patient shown in Figure 2-29.*

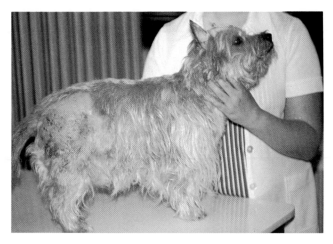

Figure 2-31 *Flea allergic Cairn Terrier with self-induced alopecia, and bacterial dermatitis on rump.*

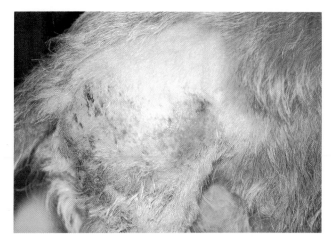

Figure 2-32 *Closer view of lesions shown in Figure 2-31.*

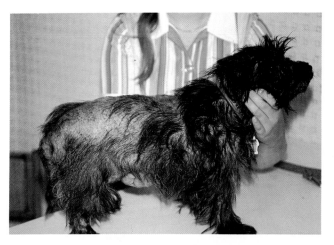

Figure 2-33 *Six-year-old Scottish Terrier with flea bite hypersensitivity. Patient's pruritus has created alopecia, erythema, and bacterial dermatitis.*

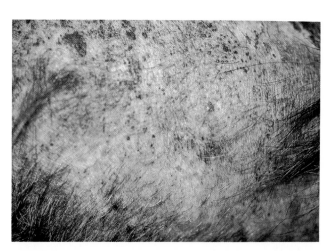

Figure 2-34 *Closer view of lesions from patient shown in Figure 2-33. Excoriations, papules, and crusts are evident.*

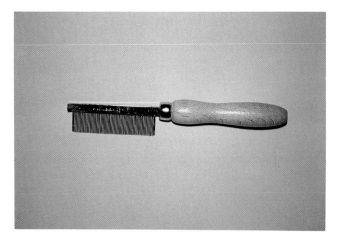

Figure 2-35 *The flea comb is essential tool in veterinary dermatology. Great aid in finding fleas and flea excreta and recommended for use in every pruritic patient.*

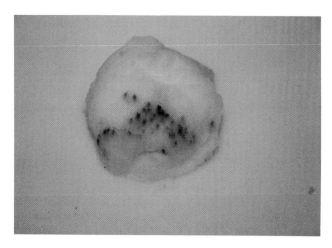

Figure 2-36 *Since fleas spend most of their life cycle off host, it is important to carefully look for flea excreta. Wetting excreta with water will produce rust-colored tinge on cotton that helps to differentiate excreta from other debris.*

Feline Flea Bite Hypersensitivity

CLINICAL SIGNS

1. Miliary dermatitis
2. Self-induced alopecia of rump, tail, and/or rear legs
3. Head and neck pruritus that typically results in excoriations
4. Eosinophilic plaque lesions usually located on the abdomen and/or medial thighs

DIFFERENTIAL DIAGNOSIS

1. Allergic inhalant disease (atopy)
2. Food hypersensitivity
3. Cheyletiella dermatitis
4. Notoedric mange
5. Dermatophyte infection
6. *Otodectes cynotis* (ear mites)

DIAGNOSTIC AIDS

1. Finding fleas and/or flea excreta on patient (always use flea comb)
2. Positive reaction to intradermally injected flea antigen
3. Response to flea eradication program

COMMENTS

Flea bite hypersensitivity is the most common form of allergic skin disease seen in the cat. Miliary dermatitis is the most common presenting sign. No breed or sex predilection exists. The average age at onset of clinical signs is 2 to 6 years of age. Since cats are such meticulous groomers, it may be impossible to find evidence of flea infestation on a cat suffering from flea bite hypersensitivity. For this reason, an important diagnostic aid in allergic feline patients is response to appropriate flea control.

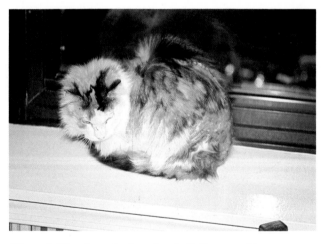

Figure 2-37   *Severely flea allergic Calico cat with self-induced lesions on rump.*

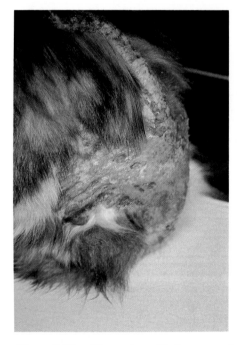

Figure 2-38   *Closer view of lesions on patient shown in Figure 2-37. Extensive self-induced erosions and ulcerations are quite evident.*

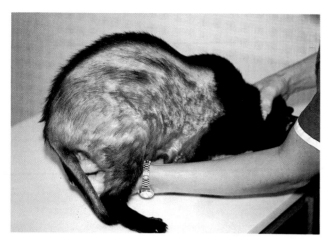

Figure 2-39 *Extensive self-induced alopecia on right side of 9-year-old mixed-breed cat with flea bite hypersensitivity.*

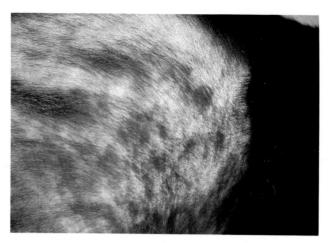

Figure 2-40 *Closer view of alopecic area on patient in Figure 2-39. Short and stubbled hairs help to differentiate self-induced alopecia from endocrine alopecia.*

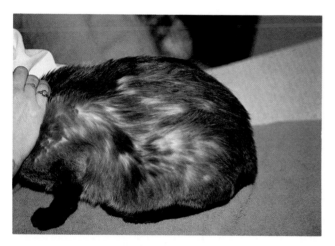

Figure 2-41 *Self-induced patchy alopecia on trunk of Siamese cat with flea bite hypersensitivity.*

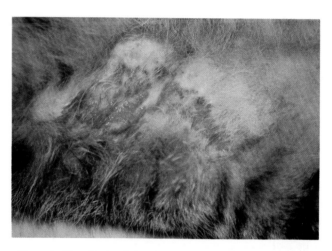

Figure 2-42 *Eosinophilic plaque on abdominal area of flea allergic feline. Lesion was created by constant licking of area.*

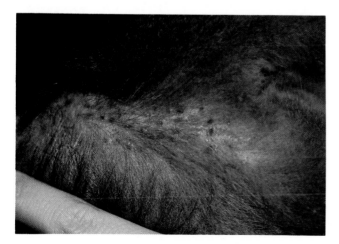

Figure 2-43 *Excoriated papules (miliary dermatitis) on midback of 2-year-old cat with flea bite allergies.*

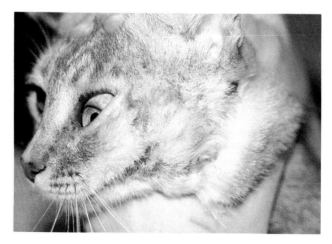

Figure 2-44 *Excoriations on face and neck of flea allergic feline. Head and neck pruritus is seen commonly in cats with hypersensitivities to flea bites, foods, and inhaled allergens.*

Canine Food Hypersensitivity

CLINICAL SIGNS

1. Nonseasonal pruritus
2. The ventrum, perineal area, and rump are most frequently involved
3. Otitis externa
4. Alopecia, erythema, lichenification, and hyperpigmentation are common sequelae to chronic pruritus
5. Secondary bacterial dermatitis
6. Secondary seborrheic dermatoses

DIFFERENTIAL DIAGNOSIS

1. Allergic inhalant disease (atopy)
2. Flea bite hypersensitivity
3. Intestinal parasite hypersensitivity
4. Hormonal hypersensitivity
5. Sarcoptic mange
6. Contact dermatitis

DIAGNOSTIC AIDS

1. Allergy test diet consisting of lamb, long-cooking rice, and distilled water for 3 to 4 weeks (The test diet must be introduced very gradually over a 7 to 10 day period to help prevent serious gastrointestinal upset.) Flavored vitamins and flavored heartworm preventative should be discontinued during the test diet.
2. Skin biopsies for histopathologic examination are not diagnostic
3. In vitro testing such as Radio-Allergo Sorbent Test (RAST) and Enzyme-Linked Immuno-Sorbent (ELISA) are considered to be less accurate than the allergy test diet

COMMENTS

Food hypersensitivity is an uncommon cause of pruritus and otitis in the dog. There is no breed or sex predilection. Young animals may be predisposed; but, the hypersensitivity to foods can develop at any age even if the patient has been eating the same diet for years. The pruritus is nonseasonal and may be poorly responsive to glucocorticoids.

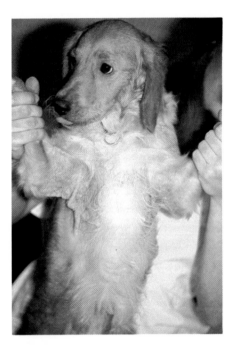

Figure 2-45   *One-year-old mixed Golden Retriever with 8-month history of pruritus involving ears, axillary, inguinal, and perianal areas. Note erythema with some hyperpigmentation of axillae.*

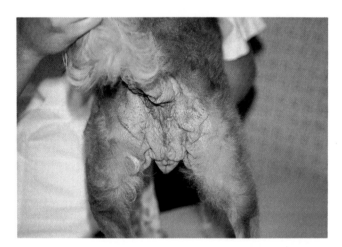

Figure 2-46   *Self-induced alopecia with erythema and hyperpigmentation of perianal and perivulvar areas of food allergic patient shown in Figure 2-45.*

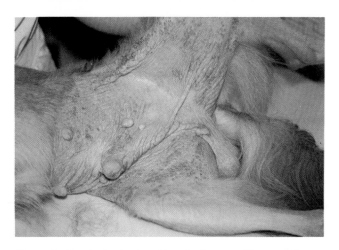

Figure 2-47 *Abdominal and inguinal areas of 2-year-old mixed-breed dog with food hypersensitivity. Note extensive self-induced alopecia, erythema, and excoriations.*

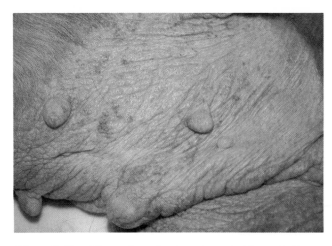

Figure 2-48 *Closer view of patient shown in Figure 2-47. Only other areas of involvement were external ear canals.*

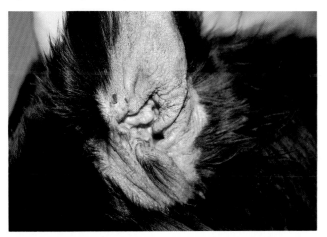

Figure 2-49 *Seborrheic otitis externa with hyperpigmentation in a 6-year-old mixed-breed dog with a 4-year history of nonseasonal pruritus and otitis.*

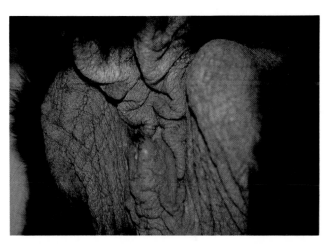

Figure 2-50 *Abdominal and inguinal areas of patient shown in Figure 2-49. Severe hyperpigmentation and lichenification are secondary to chronic licking and chewing of the area.*

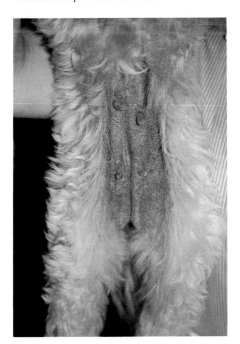

Figure 2-51 *Abdominal area of 10-year-old mixed-breed dog with 1-year history of nonseasonal pruritus involving abdominal and perianal areas.*

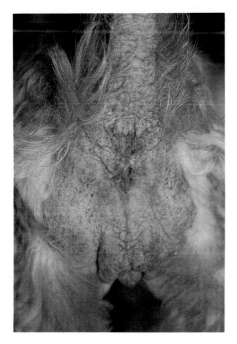

Figure 2-52 *Perianal and perivulvar areas of patient shown in Figure 2-51. Chronic pruritus has led to secondary hyperpigmentation and lichenification.*

Feline Food Hypersensitivity

CLINICAL SIGNS

1. Self-induced alopecia
2. Head and neck pruritus
3. Eosinophilic plaque lesions
4. Miliary dermatitis

DIFFERENTIAL DIAGNOSIS

1. Allergic inhalant disease (atopy)
2. Flea bite hypersensitivity
3. Psychogenic alopecia
4. Contact dermatitis
5. Dermatophyte infection
6. Cheyletiella dermatitis
7. Notoedric mange
8. *Otodectes cynotis* (ear mites)

DIAGNOSTIC AIDS

1. Allergy test diet consisting of lamb baby food and distilled water for 3 to 4 weeks. The test diet must be introduced very gradually over a 7 to 10 day period to help prevent serious gastrointestinal upsets. The test diet should not be continued for greater than 4 weeks, as serious, life-threatening dietary deficiencies may result.
2. Skin biopsies for histopathologic examination are helpful to rule out differential diagnoses but are not diagnostic for food hypersensitivity.

COMMENTS

Food hypersensitivity is an uncommon cause of nonseasonal pruritus, miliary dermatitis, and eosinophilic plaques in the cat. No age, breed, or sex predilections have been documented. Food hypersensitivity may develop in a patient even if no dietary changes have been made and the same diet has been eaten for years. The pruritus associated with food hypersensitivity may be less responsive to corticosteroids than pruritus associated with other hypersensitivities.

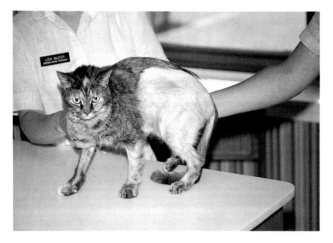

Figure 2-53 *Domestic Short-Haired cat with self-induced alopecia of legs and trunk. Patient had been food allergic for more than 2 years.*

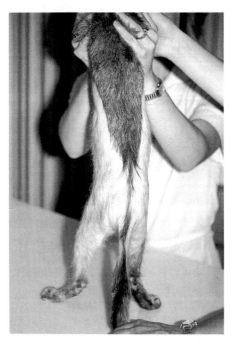

Figure 2-54 *Rear view of patient shown in Figure 2-53. Remaining hair on trunk is in areas that patient was unable to reach and lick off.*

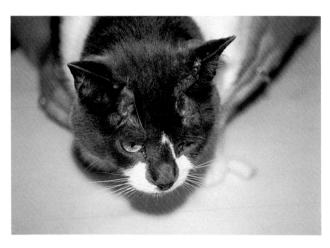

Figure 2-55   *Excoriations on face of 3-year-old food hypersensitive cat. No other lesions were present.*

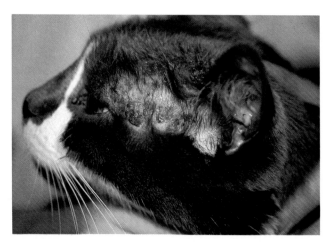

Figure 2-56   *Closer view of excoriated area on patient shown in Figure 2-55.*

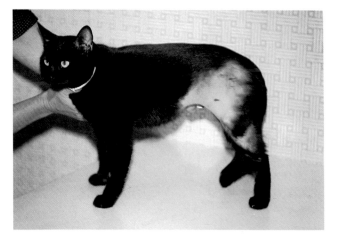

Figure 2-57   *Seven-year-old Domestic Short-Haired cat with 6-month history of pruritus caused by food hypersensitivity. Self-induced alopecia is evident on left flank and rear leg.*

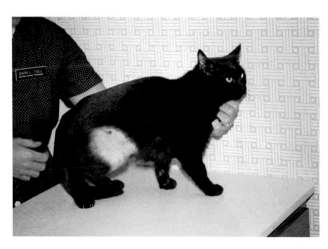

Figure 2-58   *Right side of patient shown in Figure 2-57. Areas of alopecia are bilaterally symmetric.*

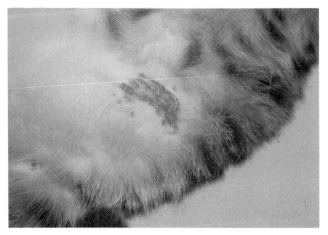

Figure 2-59   *Eosinophilic plaque on abdominal area of 2-year-old cat. Underlying etiology of this self-induced lesion was food hypersensitivity.*

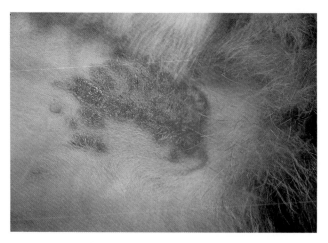

Figure 2-60   *Closer view of lesion shown in Figure 2-59.*

Allergic Contact Dermatitis

CLINICAL SIGNS

1. Pruritus involving sparsely haired "contact" areas such as chest, inguinal area, perivulvar area, perianal area, and feet
2. Allergic contact dermatitis to topical medications can occur in any area of the body; however, the external ear canal may be the most common site
3. Reactions to plastic or rubber food and water dishes, and toys are usually confined to the muzzle
4. Chronic pruritus may result in alopecia, erythema, hyperpigmentation, lichenification, seborrheic disorders and/or bacterial dermatitis

DIFFERENTIAL DIAGNOSIS

1. Allergic inhalant disease (atopy)
2. Food hypersensitivity
3. Flea bite hypersensitivity
4. Irritant contact dermatitis
5. Sarcoptic mange
6. Hookworm dermatitis
7. Bacterial folliculitis
8. Seborrheic dermatitis

DIAGNOSTIC AIDS

1. History of contact with potential contact allergen
2. Skin biopsies for histopathologic examination are usually nondiagnostic
3. Response to removal of and rechallenge with potential contact allergen
4. Patch testing (usually not practical)

COMMENTS

True allergic contact dermatitis is uncommon in the dog and cat. No age, breed, or sex predilection exists. Substances reported to cause allergic contact dermatitis include poison ivy and oak, pollens, resins, shampoos (especially tar based), insecticides, topical medications such as neomycin, wool fibers, nylon fibers, dyes, cat litter, rubber and plastic products, cleansers, and detergents.

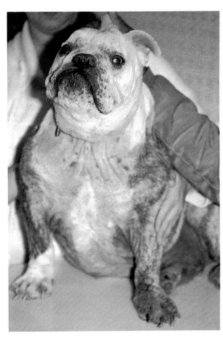

Figure 2-61 *Five-year-old English Bulldog with allergic contact dermatitis. Offending allergen was found to be sprinkle on carpet fresheners.*

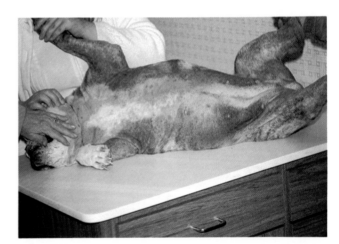

Figure 2-62 *Another view of allergic patient shown in Figure 2-61. Extensive self-induced alopecia with erythema and some hyperpigmentation is seen.*

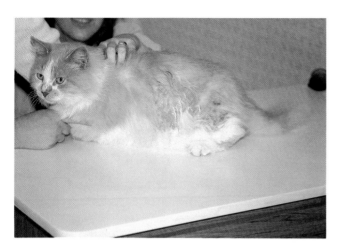

Figure 2-63 *Eight-year-old cat with allergic contact reaction to neomycin-containing ointment.*

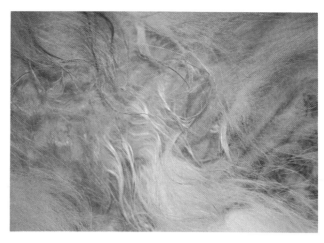

Figure 2-64 *Closer view of allergic reaction shown in Figure 2-63. Involved skin is alopecic, erythemic, edematous, and in some areas ulcerated.*

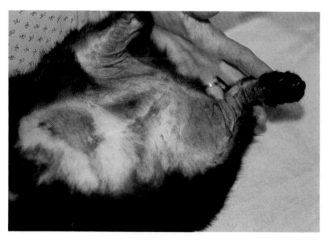

Figure 2-65 *Abdominal and inguinal areas of cat with allergic contact dermatitis. Causative allergen was found to be scented cat box litter.*

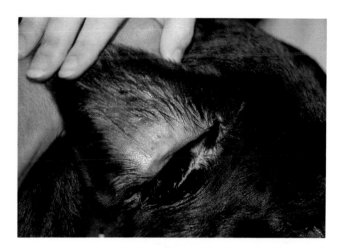

Figure 2-66 *Ear pinna of Labrador Retriever with allergic reaction to topical gentamicin. Both external ear canals and medial aspects of pinnae were erythematous and blistered.*

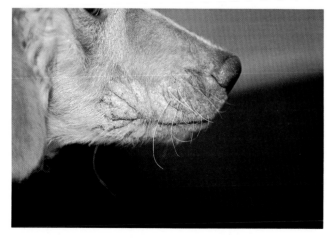

Figure 2-67 *Muzzle of patient with contact allergic reaction to rawhide chew toys. Erythema and pruritus regressed within 5 days after removal of offending allergen. Reexposure to rawhide created new lesions and pruritus within 24 hours.*

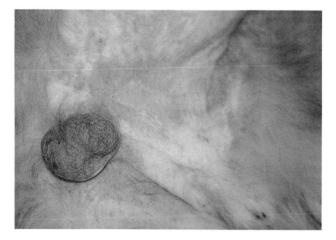

Figure 2-68 *Allergic contact dermatitis in Keeshond to poison ivy. This allergen was suspected after owners developed severe contact dermatitis after handling patient.*

Flea Collar Contact Dermatitis

CLINICAL SIGNS

1. Erythematous patches or an erythematous ring around the "collar" area
2. Pruritus may lead to excoriations
3. Secondary bacterial infection may be a complicating factor
4. Lesions may extend beyond the "collar" area

DIFFERENTIAL DIAGNOSIS

1. Some canine hormonal imbalances result in "collar" area alopecia with or without bacterial complications
2. Some canine seborrheic diseases are most severe on the ventral neck
3. Other causes of neck pruritus in the cat include in-halant, flea bite, and food hypersensitivities as well as ear mites and notoedric mange

DIAGNOSTIC AIDS

1. Classic appearance and location of lesions as well as the history of the patient wearing, or recently wearing a flea collar
2. Skin biopsies for histopathologic examination may be helpful but are rarely necessary

COMMENTS

Flea collar contact dermatitis has been reported in the dog and cat. Most reactions are probably irritant, but the severity of some reactions suggests an allergic contact basis. It is not certain if the irritant or allergic reaction is caused by the polyvinylchloride plastic collar or by the impregnated insecticide or both.

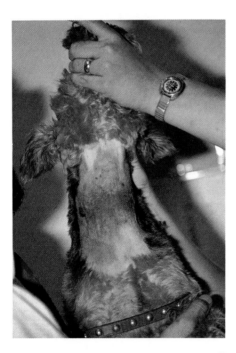

Figure 2-69 *Extensive erythema and swelling with central area of hyperpigmentation on neck of young male Welsh Terrier with flea collar contact dermatitis.*

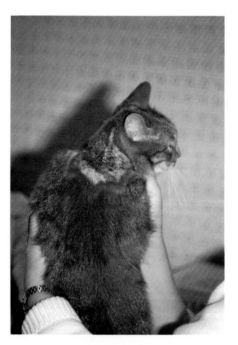

Figure 2-70 *Six-year-old mixed-breed cat shows ulcerations and excoriations on dorsal neck caused by an irritant/allergic reaction to flea collar.*

Intestinal Parasite Hypersensitivity

CLINICAL SIGNS

1. Moderate to severe pruritus is the hallmark of this disease
2. Papules and erythema may be present
3. Pruritus and/or lesions may be localized to the ventrum or may be generalized

DIFFERENTIAL DIAGNOSIS

1. Food hypersensitivity
2. Allergic inhalant disease (atopy)
3. Flea bite hypersensitivity
4. Allergic or irritant contact dermatitis
5. Bacterial folliculitis
6. Seborrheic dermatitis

DIAGNOSTIC AIDS

1. Fecal floatations
2. Response to treatment
3. Skin biopsies for histopathologic examination are not diagnostic

COMMENTS

Intestinal parasite hypersensitivity is a common cause of pruritus in the dog. It is less common in the cat. There is no age, breed, or sex predilection. Patients with other types of hypersensitivities may be predisposed. Hookworms, whipworms, ascarids, coccidia, and tapeworms have been known to cause intestinal parasite hypersensitivity, which is a Type I hypersensitivity reaction.

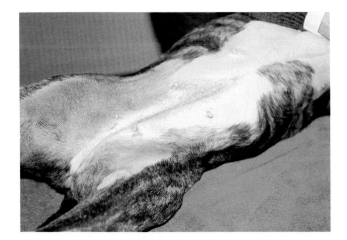

Figure 2-71 *Two-year-old Bull Terrier with several-month history of pruritus involving abdominal and inguinal areas. Treatment of patient's* Ancylostoma caninum *(hookworm) infection resulted in elimination of pruritus and dermatitis.*

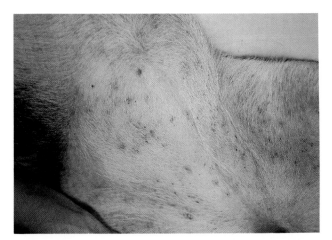

Figure 2-72 *Pruritic rash on abdomen of German Shepherd Dog with intestinal parasite hypersensitivity to* Trichuris spp. *(whipworms).*

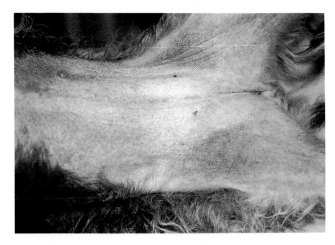

Figure 2-73 *Pruritic papular dermatitis on abdomen and medial thighs of mixed-breed dog. Patient's dermatitis was caused by hookworm* (Ancylostoma caninum) *hypersensitivity.*

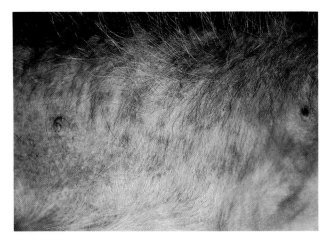

Figure 2-74 *Closer view of lesions shown in Figure 2-73.*

Hormonal Hypersensitivity

CLINICAL SIGNS

1. Pruritus usually involving the abdominal, inguinal, and perineal areas as well as medial and caudal thighs
2. Erythema and a papular eruption may develop
3. Hyperpigmentation and lichenification may be secondary to chronic pruritus
4. Lesions and pruritus have a bilaterally symmetric distribution
5. Enlargement of the nipples, mammary glands, and/or vulva

DIFFERENTIAL DIAGNOSIS

1. Flea bite hypersensitivity
2. Food hypersensitivity
3. Allergic inhalant disease (atopy)
4. Intestinal parasite hypersensitivity
5. Bacterial folliculitis
6. Allergic or irritant contact dermatitis
7. Seborrheic dermatoses

DIAGNOSTIC AIDS

1. Thorough history and physical examination
2. Intradermal skin testing with aqueous progesterone, estrogen, and testosterone
3. Response to treatment (for instance ovariohysterectomy/castration)
4. Measurement of humoral sex hormone levels is nondiagnostic

COMMENTS

Hormonal hypersensitivity is a rare cause of pruritic dermatitis in the dog. It has not been documented in the cat. There is no age or breed predilection. Most cases occur in intact female dogs. The clinical signs may initially coincide with estrus or false pregnancy. The pathomechanism may involve Type I and Type IV hypersensitivity reactions to endogenous estrogen, progesterone, and testosterone.

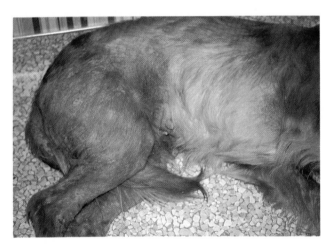

Figure 2-75 *Intact female Golden Retriever with self-induced alopecia and hyperpigmentation. Patient's skin disease was present only during pseudocyesis.*

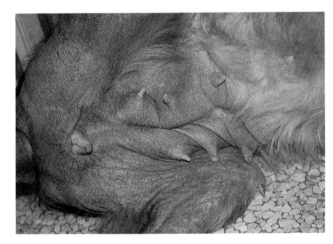

Figure 2-76 *Enlarged mammary glands of patient shown in Figure 2-75. Ovariohysterectomy was curative.*

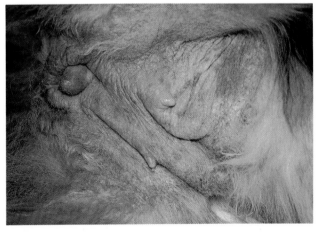

Figure 2-77 *Abdominal and inguinal areas of Shetland Sheepdog with hormonal hypersensitivity.*

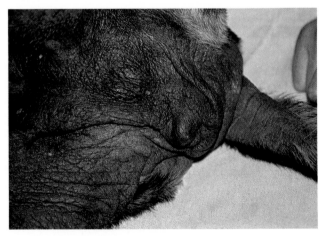

Figure 2-78 *Spayed German Shepherd Dog with pruritus and hyperpigmentation of rump and inguinal areas. Exploratory surgery revealed that an ovary remained.*

Urticaria and Angioedema (Hives)

CLINICAL SIGNS

1. Acute onset of localized or generalized wheals or edematous swellings
2. Lesions may be intensely pruritic to nonpruritic
3. Affected animals may be restless

DIFFERENTIAL DIAGNOSIS

1. Bacterial dermatitis
2. Dermatophyte infection
3. Erythema multiforme
4. Vasculitis
5. Mast cell tumor
6. Lymphoreticular neoplasia

DIAGNOSTIC AIDS

1. History of rapid onset of lesions
2. Biopsies for histopathologic examination
3. Response to treatment

COMMENTS

Urticaria and angioedema are relatively common in the dog and rare in the cat. No age, breed, or sex predilections exist. Substances reported to have caused canine or feline urticaria or angioedema include foods, drugs, insect stings, allergenic extracts, intestinal parasites, sunlight, inhaled allergens, and stress. Determining the etiology of a patient's urticaria is quite difficult in many cases.

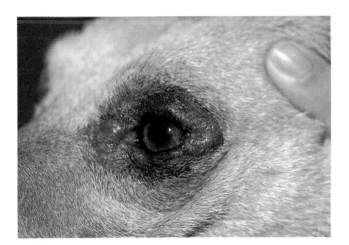

Figure 2-79   Periocular area of mixed-breed shows angioedema. Patient's acute disease was caused by a systemic reaction to intradermally injected skin test antigens.

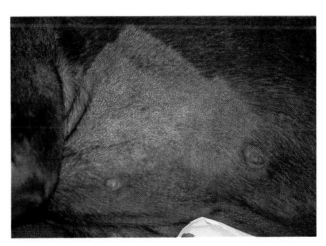

Figure 2-80   Wheals on chest of Doberman Pinscher. Patient's acute generalized urticaria was associated with intravenous administration of thyroid-stimulating hormone.

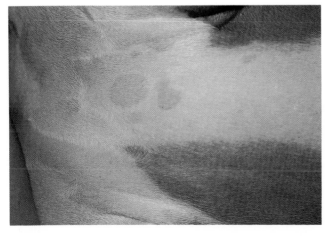

Figure 2-81   Urticarial wheals on chest of 2-year-old English Bulldog. Etiology of patient's lesions was not detected.

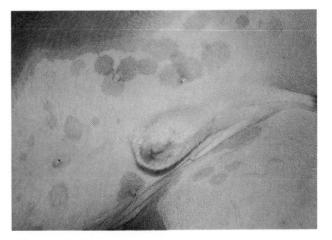

Figure 2-82   Abdominal and inguinal areas of patient shown in Figure 2-81.

Drug Eruption

CLINICAL SIGNS

1. Lesions consist of papules, macules, vesicles, petechiae, purpura, ulcers, and urticarial wheals
2. Severe erythroderma is a common finding
3. Lesions may be cutaneous and/or mucocutaneous, localized or generalized
4. The external ear canals may be involved
5. Pruritus is variable
6. Drug eruption can mimic virtually any skin disease

DIFFERENTIAL DIAGNOSIS

1. Erythema multiforme
2. Toxic epidermal necrolysis
3. Diseases of the pemphigus complex
4. Lupus erythematosus
   (*The aforementioned differentials may be drug induced.*)
5. Contact dermatitis
6. Bacterial dermatitis
7. Allergic dermatitis

DIAGNOSTIC AIDS

1. Skin biopsies for histopathologic examination may be helpful
2. History of recent exposure to a drug
3. Response to removal of suspect drug (A drug eruption may persist for months after the offending drug is discontinued.)

COMMENTS

Drug eruption is uncommon in the dog and cat. No age, breed, or sex predilection has been documented. Drug eruption is difficult to diagnose, because the lesions may resemble those of any dermatologic disorder. The lesions are usually poorly responsive to glucocorticoids. Antibiotics are the class of drugs that most frequently cause drug eruptions. However, virtually any drug may be capable of producing a drug eruption in any given patient. Routes of drug administration include oral, topical, injectable, and inhaled.

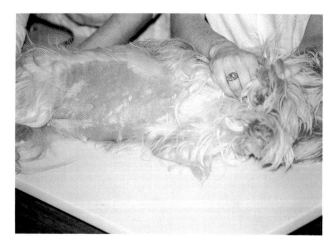

Figure 2-83   Severe ventral erythroderma associated with use of cephalosporin antibiotic.

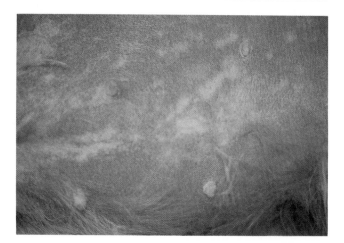

Figure 2-84   Abdomen of patient shown in Figure 2-83. Lesions were mildly pruritic.

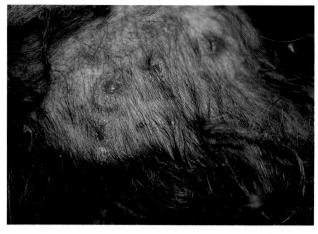

Figure 2-85   Vesicles, papules, and wheals on medial thigh of Scottish Terrier. Lesions were associated with oral lincomycin.

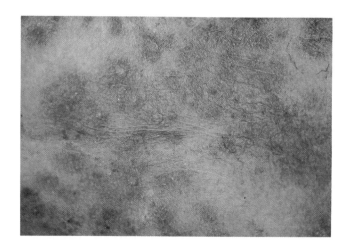

Figure 2-86   Abdomen of Old English Sheepdog shows pustules, papules, and macules associated with use of tetracycline.

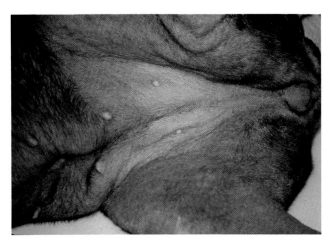

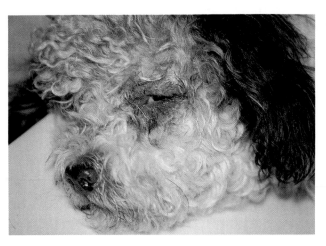

Figure 2-87 *Marked erythroderma of abdominal and inguinal areas of Doberman Pinscher. Cutaneous lesions developed 10 days after initiation of griseofulvin therapy.*

Figure 2-88 *Five-year-old Poodle with depigmentation and ulceration of nose and periocular areas. Lesions developed 72 hours after administration of DHLP vaccinations. Patient had similar, less severe reaction previous year to same vaccination.*

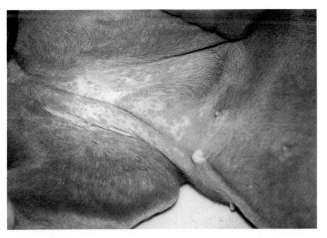

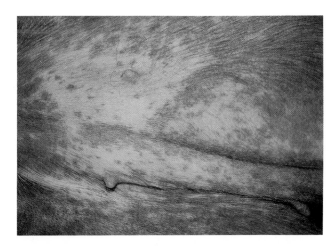

Figure 2-89 *Abdominal area of Weimariner shows marked erythroderma, macules, and papules. Lesions developed within 24 hours after a penicillin injection.*

Figure 2-90 *Closer view of patient's abdomen shown in Figure 2-89.*

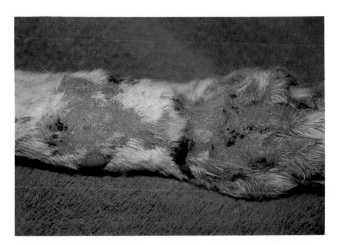

Figure 2-91 *Foreleg of 4-year-old mixed-breed dog. Leg had been injected with cobra venom to treat acral pruritic nodules. Entire leg was edematous and erythematous, with numerous areas of cutaneous necrosis.*

True Bacterial Hypersensitivity (Staphylococcal Hypersensitivity)

CLINICAL SIGNS

1. The most classical lesions are erythematous pustules or hemorrhagic bullae
2. Lesions are intensely pruritic
3. Lesions may occur in conjunction with other skin diseases

DIFFERENTIAL DIAGNOSIS

1. Bacterial folliculitis
2. Bacterial hypersensitivity-like dermatitis
3. Sarcoptic mange
4. Seborrheic dermatitis
5. Allergic inhalant disease (atopy)
6. Flea bite hypersensitivity
7. Food hypersensitivity
8. Pemphigus foliaceus
9. Demodicosis

DIAGNOSTIC AIDS

1. Bacterial cultures typically grow pure cultures of *Staphylococcus intermedius*
2. Skin biopsies for histopathologic examination are often diagnostic
3. Patients with a true bacterial hypersensitivity develop a delayed (24- to 72-hour) reaction after intradermally injected staphylococcal cell wall–toxoid product. All dogs (even normal ones) will develop an immediate wheal-and-flare reaction

COMMENTS

True bacterial hypersensitivity dermatitis is a type III hypersensitivity reaction against staphylococcal antigens. It is relatively rare in the dog and has not been reported in the cat. A hallmark of the disease is intense pruritus.

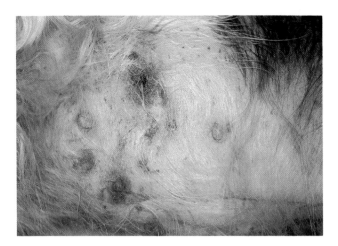

Figure 2-92 *Hemorrhagic bullae on abdomen of 8-year-old English Springer Spaniel with staphylococcal hypersensitivity.*

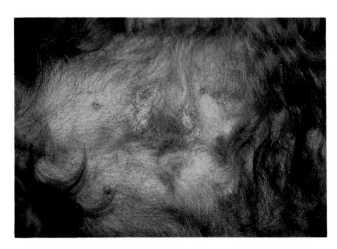

Figure 2-93 *Abdominal area of 5-year-old Poodle shows seborrheic patch with markedly erythematous border.*

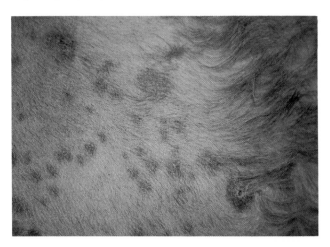

Figure 2-94 *Numerous pustules with some bullae on lateral thorax of mixed-breed dog. Patient also suffered from allergic inhalant disease.*

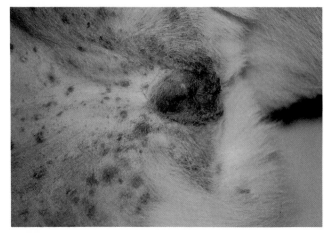

Figure 2-95 *Inguinal area of 1-year-old Akita with many hemorrhagic bullae. Patient was also hypothyroid which may have intensified bacterial hypersensitivity.*

IMMUNE-MEDIATED DERMATOSES

Erythema multiforme

Toxic epidermal necrolysis

Vogt-Koyanagi-Harada-like syndrome

Cutaneous vasculitis

Linear IgA dermatosis

Alopecia areata

Sterile nodular panniculitis

Juvenile pyoderma (juvenile cellulitis, puppy strangles)

Erythema Multiforme

CLINICAL SIGNS

1. "Target" lesions are a common finding. (Erythematous macules or plaques with blanched out or ulcerated centers)
2. Vesicles, bullae, erosions, and ulcers may also be seen
3. Lesions occur on the skin and/or mucocutaneous junctions
4. Patients rarely show signs of systemic illness

DIFFERENTIAL DIAGNOSIS

1. Urticaria
2. Pustular dermatitis
3. True bacterial hypersensitivity
4. Dermatophyte infection
5. Demodicosis

DIAGNOSTIC AIDS

1. Skin biopsies for histopathologic examination reveals hydropic interface dermatitis with single cell necrosis of keratinocytes and dermal edema; full-thickness coagulation necrosis of the epidermis
2. Biopsies for direct immunofluorescence are negative
3. Antinuclear antibody (ANA) test is negative

COMMENTS

Erythema multiforme is a rare cutaneous disease that has been reported in the dog and cat. There is no age, breed, or sex predilection. There is controversy over the pathogenesis of this disease and some researchers believe that it is not a true immune-mediated disease. Erythema multiforme has been associated with the administration of numerous drugs and underlying disease states. In many cases it is a self-limiting disease.

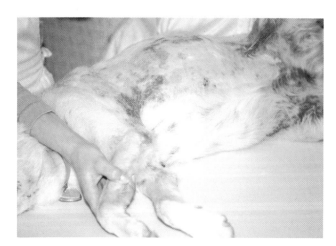

Figure 3-1   *Eleven-year-old yellow Labrador Retriever has coalescing, erythematous lesions that involve entire trunk. Lesions were nonpruritic.*

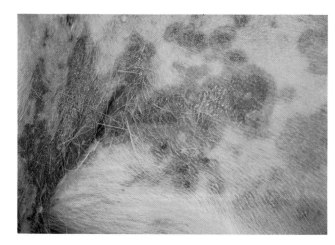

Figure 3-2   *Closer view of "target" lesions in axillary area of patient shown in Figure 3-1.*

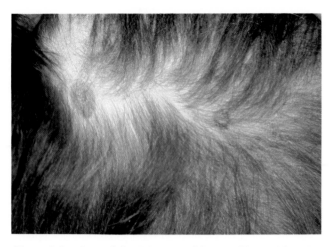

Figure 3-3   *Lateral thoracic area of 3-year-old mixed-breed dog with erythema multiforme. "Target" lesions are erythematous, somewhat circular, and have pale centers.*

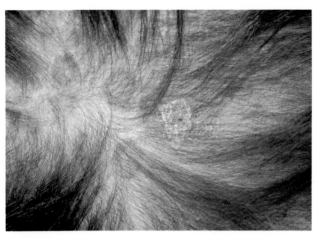

Figure 3-4   *Lesions on ventral thoracic area of patient shown in Figure 3-3.*

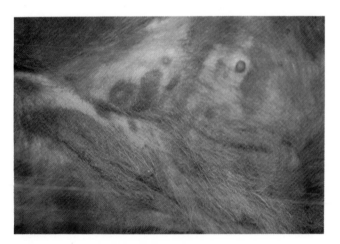

Figure 3-5   *Abdomen of Golden Retriever shows erythema multiforme. This patient's disease was associated with administration of cephalosporin antibiotics.*

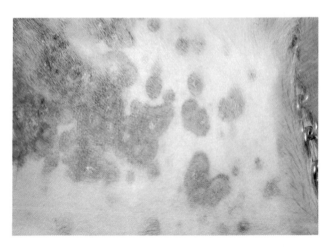

Figure 3-6   *Right shoulder area of 6-year-old Akita. Patient's erythema multiforme was caused by adverse reaction to gold salt therapy for pemphigus foliaceus.*

Toxic Epidermal Necrolysis

CLINICAL SIGNS

1. Lesions include erythema, vesicles, epidermal collarettes, erosions, and ulcers
2. Lesions occur on skin, mucocutaneous junctions, and/or footpads
3. Patients frequently show signs of systemic illness such as fever, depression, and anorexia
4. Lesions typically are painful and mildly to nonpruritic

DIFFERENTIAL DIAGNOSIS

1. Erythema multiforme
2. Pemphigus vulgaris
3. Bullous pemphigoid
4. Systemic lupus erythematosus
5. Lymphoreticular neoplasia

DIAGNOSTIC AIDS

1. Skin biopsies for histopathologic examination reveals hydropic interface dermatitis and full-thickness coagulation necrosis of the epidermis.
2. Biopsies for direct immunofluorescence testing are negative
3. Antinuclear antibody (ANA) test is negative
4. History of recent drug administration
5. CBC, chemistry profile and blood cultures to search for presence of underlying disease state

COMMENTS

Toxic epidermal necrolysis is a rare, serious, life-threatening disease that has been reported in the dog and cat. No age, breed, or sex predilection exists. "Toxic epidermal necrolysis" may simply be a more serious form of erythema multiforme. As with erythema multiforme, there is controversy over the pathogenesis and some researchers believe that it is not an immune-mediated disease. Possible causes include drugs, bacterial endocarditis, neoplastic disease, and idiopathic disease.

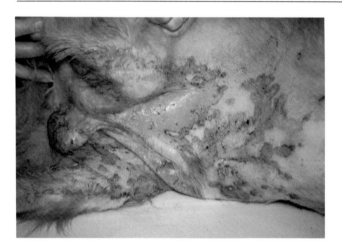

Figure 3-7   *Severe ulceration on abdomen and groin of 7-year-old dog with toxic epidermal necrolysis. Patient's disease was possibly caused by cephalosporin antibiotics.*

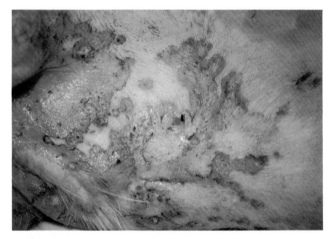

Figure 3-8   *Closer view of serpiginous ulcerations shown in Figure 3-7.*

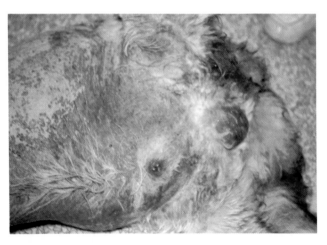

Figure 3-9   *Severely ulcerated ventrum of 13-year-old German Shepherd Dog. Lesions developed while patient was receiving gold salt injections.*

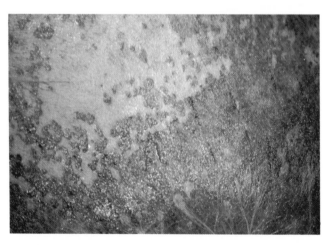

Figure 3-10   *Closer view of lesions shown in Figure 3-9. (Photographs were taken minutes after patient died.)*

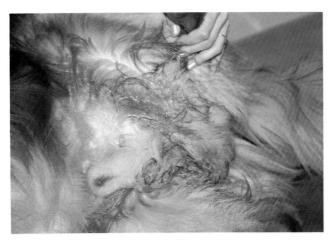

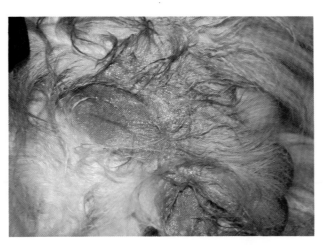

Figure 3-11 *Two-year-old Golden Retriever with toxic epidermal necrolysis. Ulcerative lesions in groin developed within 14 days after initiation of treatment with thyroid hormone supplementation.*

Figure 3-12 *Closer view of lesions shown in Figure 3-11. Lesions healed soon after withdrawal of L-thyroxine. Because of potential life-threatening nature of toxic epidermal necrolysis, challenge with T_4 was never attempted.*

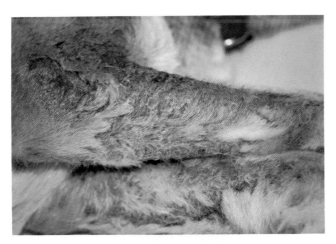

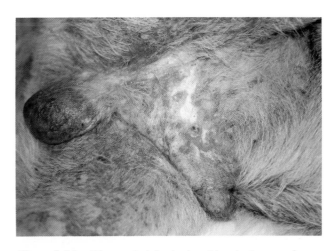

Figure 3-13 *Severely ulcerated forelegs of 3-year-old dog with toxic epidermal necrolysis. Lesions developed while patient was receiving trimethoprim-sulfa antibiotic for treatment of lacerations.*

Figure 3-14 *Ulcerated abdominal and inguinal areas of patient shown in Figure 3-13. Patient died 5 days after photographs were taken.*

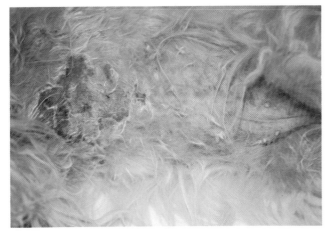

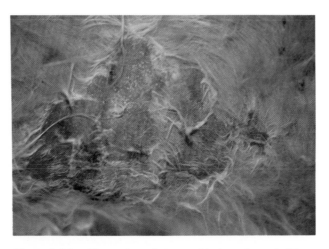

Figure 3-15 *Ulcerated and erythematous lesions on thorax and abdomen of 13-year-old Maltese. Underlying etiology of patient's toxic epidermal necrolysis was not detected.*

Figure 3-16 *Closer view of ulcerated lesions shown in Figure 3-15.*

Vogt-Koyanagi-Harada-like Syndrome

CLINICAL SIGNS

1. Hypopigmentation and/or depigmentation (vitiligo) of nose, lips, eyelids, anus, and/or footpads
2. Involved areas may become ulcerated
3. Depigmentation of hair (poliosis) may be seen
4. Bilateral uveitis

DIFFERENTIAL DIAGNOSIS

1. Acquired hypopigmentation/depigmentation due to contact irritation or idiopathic disease
2. Discoid lupus erythematosus
3. Systemic lupus erythematosus
4. Lymphoreticular neoplasia

DIAGNOSTIC AIDS

1. Skin biopsies for histopathologic examination reveals histiocytic lichenoid interface dermatitis
2. Skin biopsies for direct immunofluorescence testing are usually negative
3. Antinuclear antibody (ANA) test is negative
4. Complete ophthalmic examination

COMMENTS

Vogt-Koyanagi-Harada-like syndrome is a rare disease of the dog. There is no known age or sex predilection. Akitas, Samoyeds, and Chow Chows are predisposed. The uveitis that is associated with the disease may lead to blindness.

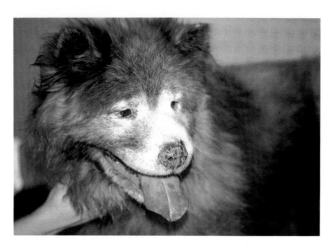

Figure 3-17   *Five-year-old Chow Chow with hypopigmentation and depigmentation of nose, tongue, lips and periocular areas. Generalized depigmentation of hair (poliosis) has also occurred.*

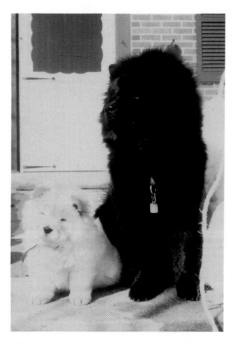

Figure 3-19   *Adult black Chow Chow is patient pictured in Figures 3-17 and 3-18 before onset of depigmentation caused by Vogt-Koyanagi-Harada-like syndrome.*

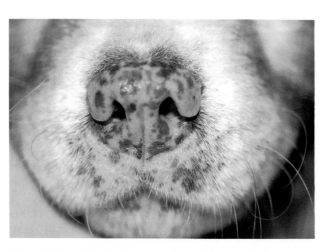

Figure 3-18   *Muzzle of patient shown in Figure 3-17.*

Cutaneous Vasculitis

CLINICAL SIGNS

1. Lesions include erythema, purpura, ulcerations, and necrosis
2. Lesions typically involve the ear pinnae, oral cavity, mucocutaneous junctions, and/or footpads
3. Signs of systemic illness may be present

DIFFERENTIAL DIAGNOSIS

1. Frostbite
2. Cold agglutinin disease
3. Systemic lupus erythematosus
4. Disseminated intravascular coagulation

DIAGNOSTIC AIDS

1. Skin biopsies for histopathologic examination reveals leukocytoclastic vasculitis
2. Biopsies for direct immunofluorescence are usually positive
3. Antinuclear antibody (ANA) test is negative

COMMENTS

Cutaneous vasculitis is an uncommon disease of the dog and cat. There is no age or sex predilection. Reported causes include chemicals, drugs, various infections, systemic lupus erythematosus, Rocky Mountain spotted fever, malignancy, and idiopathic disease. Not all cases of cutaneous vasculitis are immune-mediated.

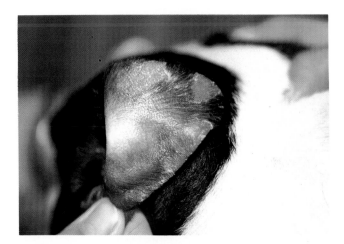

Figure 3-20   *Medial aspect of ear pinna of Boston Terrier. Note marked erythema of pinna, with alopecia and scaling of margins.*

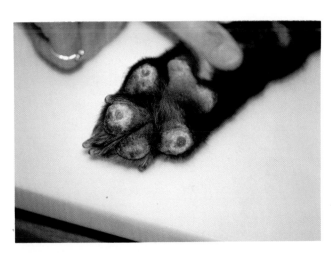

Figure 3-21   *Footpads of patient shown in Figure 3-20 show central ulceration covered by crusts.*

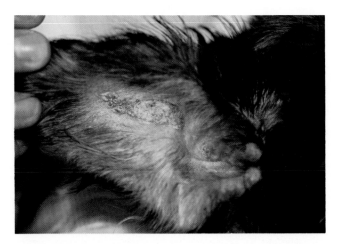

Figure 3-22   *Medial aspect of ear pinna of 8-year-old dog shows erythema, ulceration, and crusting which follow vascular channel.*

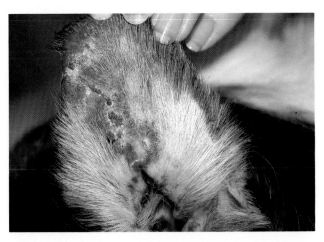

Figure 3-23   *Mixed-breed dog shows hyperpigmentation and crusts along vascular channel of medial aspect of ear pinna.*

Linear IgA Dermatosis

CLINICAL SIGNS

1. The classic lesion is a sterile subcorneal pustule
2. Alopecia, scaling, and crusting are common
3. Lesions are found most frequently on the trunk
4. Pruritus is mild to nonexistent

DIFFERENTIAL DIAGNOSIS

1. Bacterial folliculitis
2. Pemphigus foliaceus
3. Subcorneal pustular dermatosis
4. Systemic lupus erythematosus
5. Demodicosis
6. Dermatophyte infection

DIAGNOSTIC AIDS

1. Skin biopsies for histopathologic examination reveals subcorneal pustular dermatitis
2. Biopsies for direct immunofluorescence are positive for IgA and possibly C3
3. Antinuclear antibody (ANA) test is negative

COMMENTS

Linear IgA dermatosis is a rare immune-mediated disease that has been reported only in adult Short-Haired Dachshunds of both sexes. Affected dogs do not show signs of systemic illness. The underlying etiology is not known.

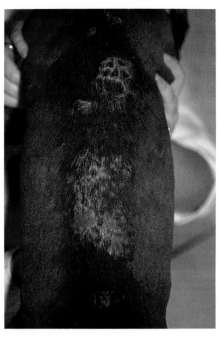

Figure 3-24   *Alopecia, scaling, and crusting on back of Short-Haired Dachshund with linear IgA dermatosis.*

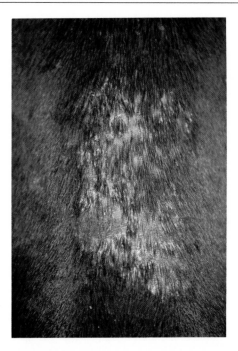

Figure 3-25   *Closer view of lesions shown in Figure 3-24. Original pustules were soon replaced by alopecia and crusts.*

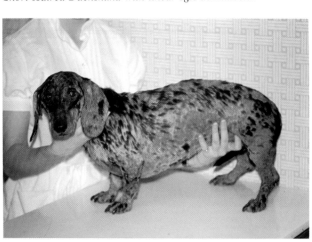

Figure 3-26   *Standard Short-Haired Dachshund has generalized alopecia with few patches of hair remaining.*

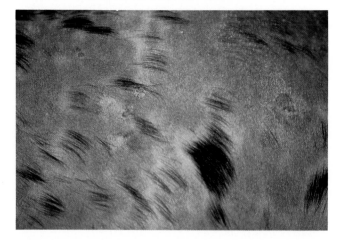

Figure 3-27   *Closer view of lesions shown in Figure 3-26. Subcorneal pustule is still evident in patient's advanced disease.*

Alopecia Areata

CLINICAL SIGNS

1. Focal or multifocal areas of alopecia
2. Skin in involved areas frequently becomes hyperpigmented
3. Patients are not pruritic

DIFFERENTIAL DIAGNOSIS

1. Demodicosis
2. Dermatophyte infection
3. Bacterial folliculitis
4. Various endocrinopathies
5. Injection reactions

DIAGNOSTIC AIDS

1. Skin biopsies for histopathologic examination reveals the accumulation of mononuclear cells around the inferior segment of anagen hair bulbs
2. Biopsies for direct immunofluorescence are usually, negative

COMMENTS

Alopecia areata is a rare disease that has been reported in the dog and cat. There is no known age, breed, or sex predilection. The cause is not known but is thought to be immune mediated.

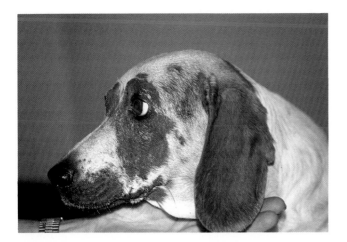

Figure 3-28 *Face of 8-year-old mixed Beagle with alopecia areata. Note marked periocular and muzzle alopecia with hyperpigmentation.*

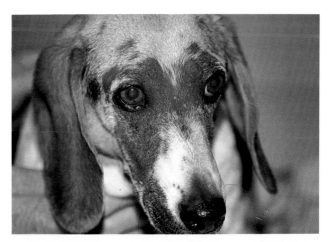

Figure 3-29 *Another view of patient shown in Figure 3-28. Lesions were nonpruritic and nonpainful. Other areas of body were not involved.*

Sterile Nodular Panniculitis

CLINICAL SIGNS

1. One or more subcutaneous nodules often with draining tracts
2. Nodules range from 1 to 9 cm in diameter
3. Any area of the body may be involved, but lesions are most commonly found on the ventrolateral thorax and abdomen
4. Exudate from lesions may be yellow and oily or hemopurulent
5. Signs of systemic disease such as depression, anorexia, fever, and weight loss may be seen
6. Lymphadenopathy may be present
7. Lesions often heal with depressed scars
8. Lesions are usually painful and nonpruritic

DIFFERENTIAL DIAGNOSIS

1. Neoplasia
2. Deep pyoderma
3. Various "cysts"
4. Foreign body granuloma
5. Infectious granuloma

DIAGNOSTIC AIDS

1. Excision biopsies for histopathologic examination
2. Examination of the exudate is often helpful
3. Cultures for bacteria will be negative

COMMENTS

Sterile nodular panniculitis is an uncommon disease of the dog. It is less common in the cat. No age, breed, or sex predilection has been documented. An underlying etiology for most cases of panniculitis cannot be determined.

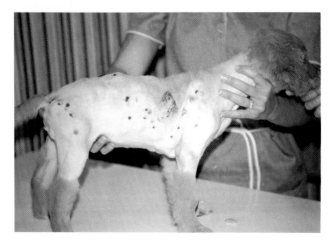

Figure 3-30 Ten-week-old Golden Retriever with numerous subcutaneous nodules. (Truncal hair was shaved.)

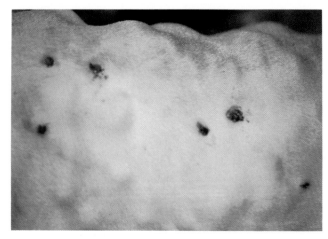

Figure 3-31 Closer view of patient in Figure 3-30. Nodules ranged in size from 1 to 5.5 cm. Many lesions were draining.

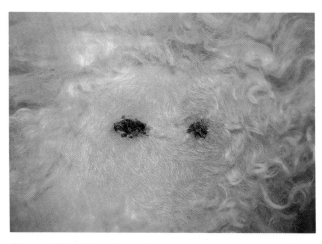

Figure 3-32 Two ulcerated panniculitis nodules on shoulder of 6-year-old male Maltese.

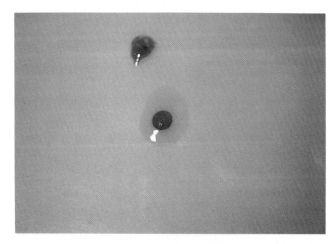

Figure 3-33 Exudate from nodules of panniculitis patient. Yellow "chicken fat" material is characteristic of this disease.

Juvenile Pyoderma (Juvenile Cellulitis, Puppy Strangles)

CLINICAL SIGNS

1. The most common clinical sign is swelling of the lips and eyelids
2. The ear pinnae are often edematous and may be ulcerated
3. Conjunctivitis and blepharitis may be present
4. The anus and prepuce or vulva may be involved
5. The submandibular lymph nodes are markedly enlarged and may rupture and drain. Other lymph nodes may also be involved
6. Puppies usually have much pain and may be anorectic, febrile, and depressed

DIFFERENTIAL DIAGNOSIS

1. Deep pyoderma
2. Demodicosis
3. Autoimmune skin disease

DIAGNOSTIC AIDS

1. Location and appearance of lesions as well as the age of the patient
2. Skin biopsies for histopathologic examination may be helpful but rarely necessary
3. Cultures for bacteria are negative unless lesions have become secondarily infected

COMMENTS

Juvenile pyoderma affects puppies between 3 and 20 weeks of age. Golden Retrievers and Dachshunds may be predisposed. No sex predilection exists. The disease is *not* caused by a bacterial infection; however, in some cases the lesions become secondarily infected by *Staphylococcus intermedius*. The etiology of this disease is not known. The author believes that it is a hypersensitivity of the immune system and in some cases is possibly induced by vaccination.

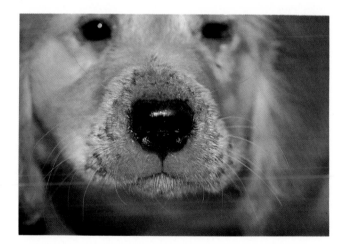

Figure 3-34 *Alopecia, erythema, pustules, and swelling on muzzle of 6-week-old Golden Retriever.*

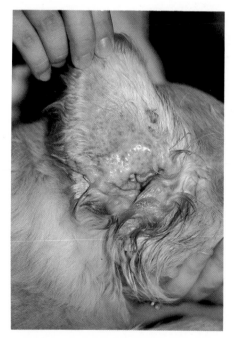

Figure 3-35 *Markedly edematous ear pinna of patient shown in Figure 3-34. Note glistening surface and serum exudate.*

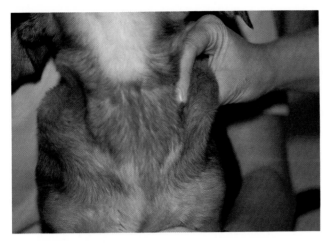

Figure 3-36 *Enlarged submandibular lymph nodes in 14-week-old mixed-breed puppy with juvenile pyoderma.*

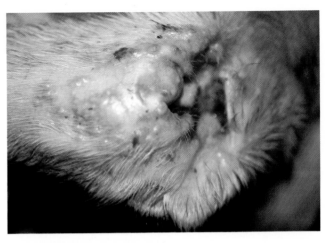

Figure 3-37 *Ear pinna of patient in Figure 3-36. Note papules, pustules, and glistening surface.*

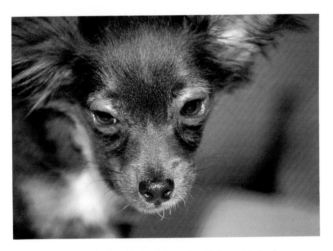

Figure 3-38 *Blepharitis in 11-week-old Long-Haired Chihuahua with juvenile pyoderma.*

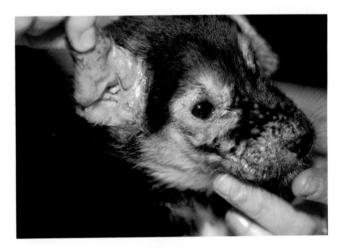

Figure 3-39 *Four-week-old mixed-breed puppy has several signs of juvenile pyoderma. Patient's lesions resulted in facial scarring.*

AUTOIMMUNE DERMATOSES

Pemphigus foliaceus

Pemphigus erythematosus

Pemphigus vulgaris

Pemphigus vegetans

Canine pemphigoid (bullous pemphigoid)

Systemic lupus erythematosus

Discoid lupus erythematosus

Cold agglutinin disease

Pemphigus Foliaceus

CLINICAL SIGNS

1. Crusts, papules, pustules, and erosions of the face, ear pinnae, and trunk
2. Hyperkeratosis of the footpads may be the only clinical sign
3. Patients with severe skin disease often show signs of systemic illness such as depression, fever, anorexia, and weight loss
4. Pruritus and pain are variable

DIFFERENTIAL DIAGNOSIS

1. Other forms of pemphigus
2. Systemic lupus erythematosus
3. Discoid lupus erythematosus
4. Zinc dermatopathy
5. Demodicosis
6. Dermatophyte infection
7. Nasal pyoderma
8. Nasal solar dermatitis
9. Bacterial folliculitis and hypersensitivity dermatitis
10. Seborrheic skin disease
11. Dermatomyositis

DIAGNOSTIC AIDS

1. Skin biopsies for histopathologic examination reveals intragranular or subcorneal cleft, vesicle, or pustule formation. (Acantholytic keratinocytes are usually present within these lesions.)
2. Biopsies for direct immunofluorescence are positive
3. Indirect immunofluorescence is negative
4. Antinuclear antibody (ANA) test is negative

COMMENTS

Pemphigus foliaceus is the most common form of autoimmune skin disease seen in the dog and cat. Lesions are often first noticed on the face and/or footpads. Lesions rarely involve the mucocutaneous junctions and oral cavity. No age or sex predilections have been reported. Short-Haired Dachshunds, Akitas, and Chow Chows may be predisposed. No breed predilection has been documented in cats.

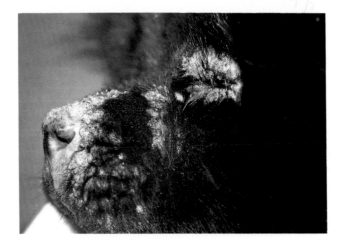

Figure 4-1 *Five-year-old Chow Chow with hypopigmentation, depigmentation, erythema, and crusting of nose, muzzle, and periocular area.*

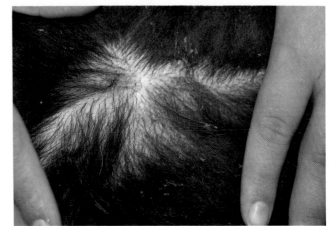

Figure 4-2 *Erythematous papules, macules, and plaques involving trunk of Chow Chow in Figure 4-1.*

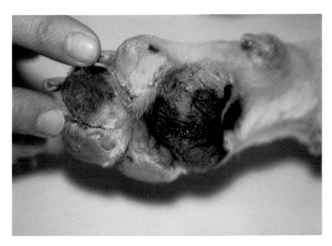

Figure 4-3 *Ulcerated, peeling footpads of 3-year-old Dalmatian with pemphigus foliaceus.*

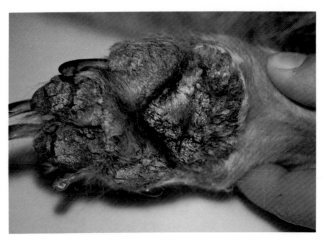

Figure 4-4 *Hyperkeratotic, cracked, and fissured footpad of 5-year-old German Shepherd Dog. Lesions were mildly pruritic and quite painful.*

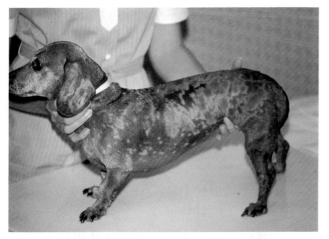

Figure 4-5 *Thirteen-year-old Miniature Short-Haired Dachshund with severe patchy, coalescing truncal alopecia and erythema. Patient had been receiving treatment for pemphigus foliaceus for 3 weeks.*

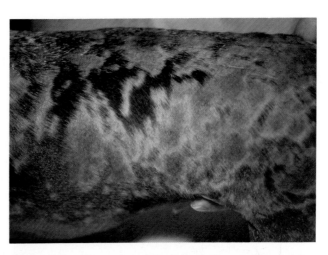

Figure 4-6 *Closer view of Dachshund shown in Figure 4-5. Note hyperpigmentation of many areas that are in healing stages.*

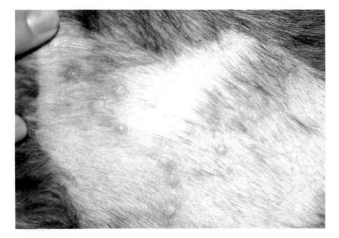

Figure 4-7 *Sterile pustules with erythematous borders on lateral thoracic area of Old English Sheepdog.*

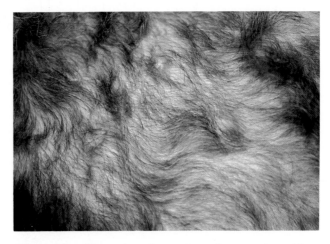

Figure 4-8 *Closer view of truncal pustules on patient with pemphigus foliaceus shown in Figure 4-7.*

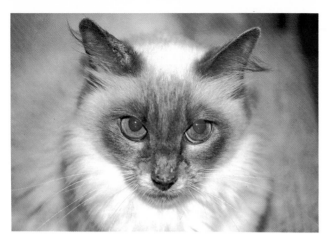

Figure 4-9   Eight-year-old cat with pemphigus foliaceus. Note alopecia, erythema, scaling, and peeling of face. Nose is slightly ulcerated, with crusts. Right ear pinna shows alopecia and crusts.

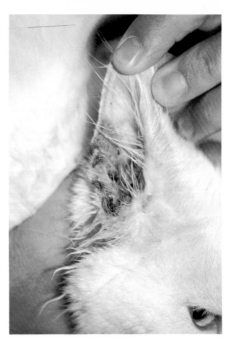

Figure 4-10   Ulcerated and crusted medial aspect of right ear pinna of Domestic Short-Haired cat with pemphigus foliaceus.

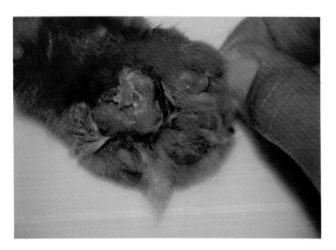

Figure 4-11   Erythematous, swollen, and peeling footpads of 6-year-old pemphigus foliaceus patient.

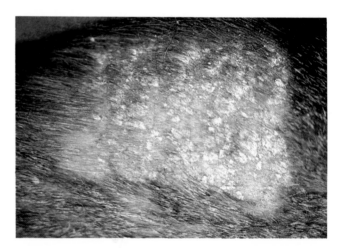

Figure 4-12   Shaved lateral thoracic area of pemphigus foliaceus patient shows extensive scale formation.

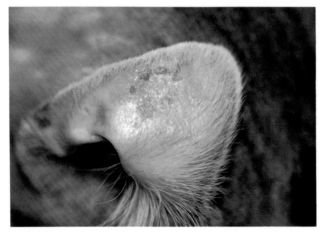

Figure 4-13   Ear pinna of mixed Siamese cat shows marked erythema and honey-colored crusts covering ruptured pustules and papules.

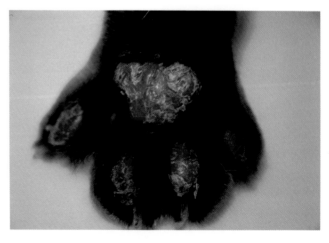

Figure 4-14   Footpads of cat shown in Figure 4-13 show scaling and peeling with area of erosion.

Pemphigus Erythematosus

CLINICAL SIGNS

1. Lesions include alopecia, erythema, scales, crusts, and ulceration
2. Lesions are almost always limited to the face and ear pinnae
3. Involvement of the feet and scrotum has been rarely reported
4. Lesions do NOT involve the oral cavity

DIFFERENTIAL DIAGNOSIS

1. Other forms of pemphigus
2. Discoid lupus erythematosus
3. Systemic lupus erythematosus
4. Nasal solar dermatitis
5. Zinc dermatopathy
6. Nasal pyoderma
7. Dermatophyte infection
8. Demodicosis
9. Dermatomyositis

DIAGNOSTIC AIDS

1. Skin biopsies for histopathologic examination reveals intragranular or subcorneal cleft, vesicle, or pustule formation. (Acantholytic keratinocytes are usually present.)
2. Biopsies for direct immunofluorescence are positive
3. Indirect immunofluorescence testing is negative
4. Antinuclear antibody (ANA) test may be positive

COMMENTS

Pemphigus erythematosus is a rare autoimmune skin disease that has been reported in the dog and cat. There is no known age or sex predilection. Collies may be predisposed. Since some patients have a positive ANA blood test and positive basement membrane zone fluorescence, it is thought that pemphigus erythematosus may be a crossover disease between pemphigus and lupus erythematosus.

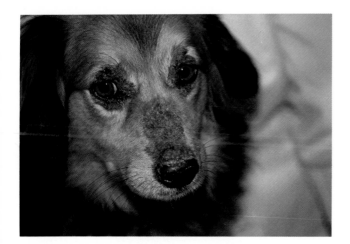

Figure 4-15 *Mixed-breed dog with alopecia and crusts on bridge of nose and periocular areas. Lesions were nonpruritic and nonpainful.*

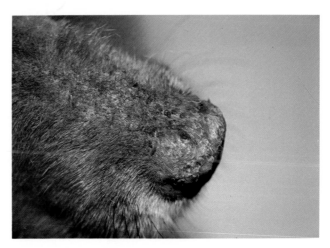

Figure 4-16 *Erythema, scales, and crusts on nose of 8-year-old mixed-breed dog with pemphigus erythematosus. No other areas of the body were involved.*

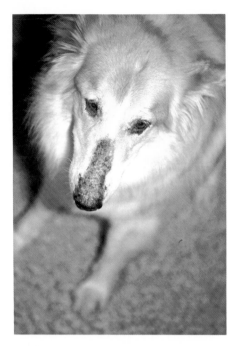

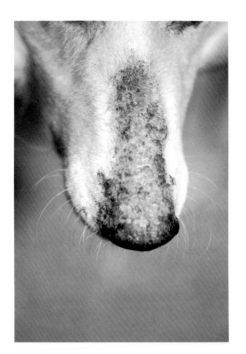

Figure 4-17   *Eleven-year-old Collie with pemphigus erythematosus. Bridge of nose is alopecic, erythematous, and crusted. Periocular areas are involved to a lesser extent.*

Figure 4-18   *Closer view of bridge of nose of patient in Figure 4-17.*

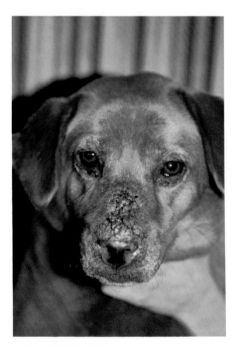

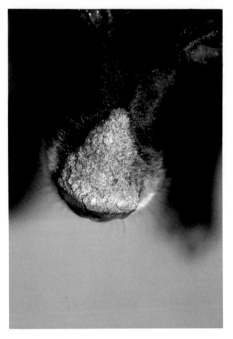

Figure 4-19   *Face of 3-year-old mixed Chow Chow with pemphigus erythematosus. Note alopecia, erythema, swelling, and crusts on bridge of nose. Nose itself is slightly hypopigmented. Periocular areas are also involved.*

Figure 4-20   *Six-year-old mixed German Shepherd Dog. Note extensive crusting on nose and bridge of nose. Periocular areas are slightly erythematous and crusted. No other lesions were present.*

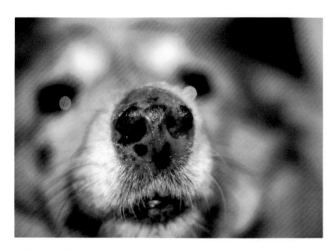

Figure 4-21 *Nose of 11-year-old Shetland Sheepdog. Note hypopigmentation, depigmentation, swelling, erythema, and erosion. This patient has no other lesions.*

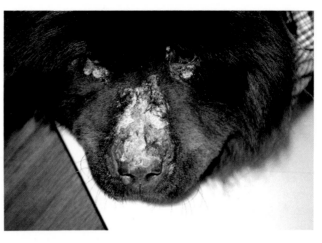

Figure 4-22 *Face of 3-year-old Chow Chow with pemphigus erythematosus. Nose is hypopigmented and bridge of nose is alopecic with erythema, scales, and crusts. Periocular lesions are also evident.*

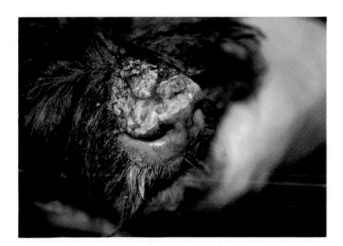

Figure 4-23 *Face of 14-year-old mixed Miniature Schnauzer with pemphigus erythematosus. Nose, nares, and nasal philtrum show hypopigmentation, erythema, erosion, and crusts.*

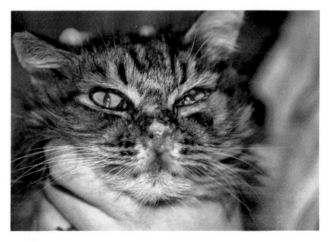

Figure 4-24 *Mixed-breed cat with pemphigus erythematosus shows facial erythema, ulcerations, and crusts.*

Pemphigus Vulgaris

CLINICAL SIGNS

1. Cutaneous and mucocutaneous lesions include erosions, ulcers, vesicles, and crusts
2. Oral cavity ulceration is frequently present
3. Paronychia may be present
4. Signs of systemic illness such as depression, fever, anorexia, and weight loss are often complicating factors
5. Pruritus and pain are variable

DIFFERENTIAL DIAGNOSIS

1. Other forms of pemphigus
2. Systemic lupus erythematosus
3. Canine pemphigoid
4. Toxic epidermal necrolysis
5. Drug eruption

6. Ulcerative stomatitis
7. Lymphoreticular neoplasia

DIAGNOSTIC AIDS

1. Skin biopsies for histopathologic examination reveals suprabasilar clefts and vesicles with acantholytic keratinocytes
2. Biopsies for direct immunofluorescence are positive
3. Direct smears from intact vesicles may show acantholytic keratinocytes
4. Indirect immunofluorescence testing is negative
5. Antinuclear antibody (ANA) test is negative

COMMENTS

Pemphigus vulgaris is a rare autoimmune skin disease that has been reported in both dogs and cats. It is the most severe form of pemphigus. There is no known age, breed, or sex predilection.

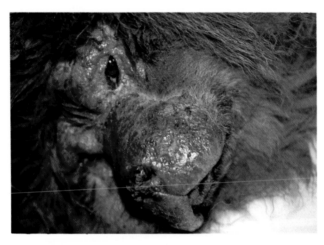

Figure 4-25 *Severely ulcerated face of 4-year-old Chow Chow with pemphigus vulgaris.*

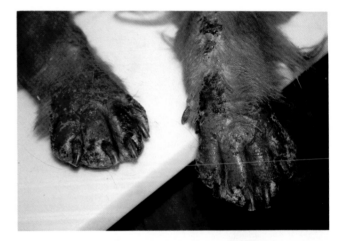

Figure 4-26 *Forefeet of Chow Chow shown in Figure 4-25.*

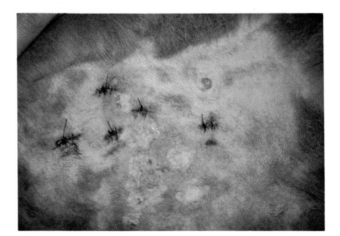

Figure 4-27 *Lateral thorax of patient shown in Figures 4-25 and 4-26. Erythematous, scaling, coalescing lesions are seen. (Note sutures at 5 biopsy sites.)*

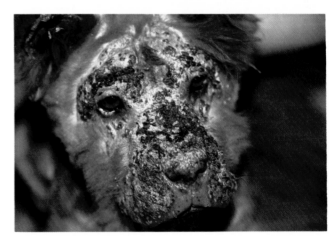

Figure 4-28 *Patient shown in Figures 4-25 to 4-27 after 3 months of treatment.*

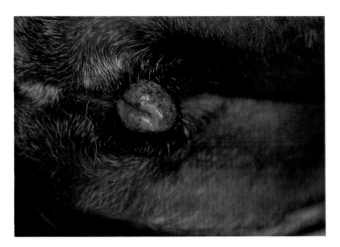

Figure 4-29 *Ulcerated vulva of 9-year-old German Short-Haired Pointer with pemphigus vulgaris. Lesions were also present on footpads and in oral cavity.*

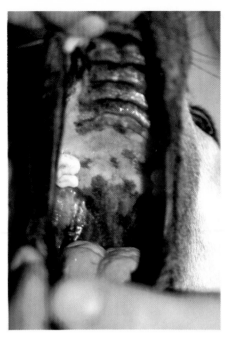

Figure 4-30 *Ulcerated hard palate of German Shepherd Dog with pemphigus vulgaris. Ulcerated lesions were also present on anus, scrotum, and prepuce.*

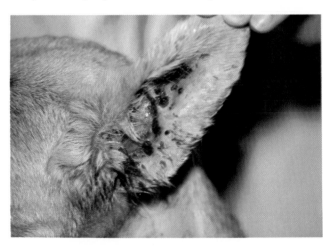

Figure 4-31 *Ear pinna of 6-year-old mixed-breed dog. Entire medial aspect of pinna is erythematous and ulcerated. Many areas are covered by serosanguinous crusts.*

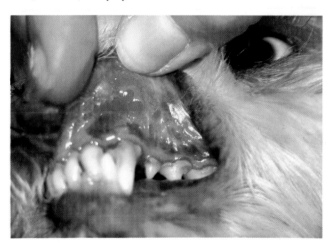

Figure 4-32 *Oral cavity of 4-year-old Cairn Terrier. Note ulceration and petechiasis of buccal mucosa.*

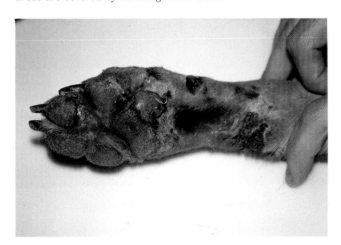

Figure 4-33 *Forefoot of Doberman Pinscher with pemphigus vulgaris. Third carpal pad and metacarpal pad are sloughing.*

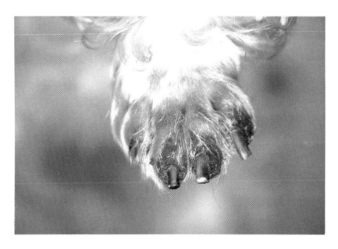

Figure 4-34 *Forefoot of West Highland White Terrier with pemphigus vulgaris. Note extensive ulceration of nail bed areas.*

Pemphigus Vegetans

CLINICAL SIGNS

1. Flat-topped, firm pustules
2. Lesions are most common in axillary and inguinal areas
3. Verrucous vegetations may be present
4. Pruritus and pain are usually absent

DIFFERENTIAL DIAGNOSIS

1. Other forms of pemphigus
2. Bacterial skin infection
3. Dermatophyte infection
4. Subcorneal pustular dermatosis
5. Cutaneous neoplasia

DIAGNOSTIC AIDS

1. Skin biopsies for histopathologic examination reveals intraepidermal microabscesses that contain mainly eosinophils and acantholytic keratinocytes
2. Biopsies for direct immunofluorescence are positive intercellular fluorescence in the epidermis
3. Antinuclear antibody (ANA) test is negative

COMMENTS

Pemphigus vegetans is the rarest form of pemphigus seen in the dog. It has not been reported in the cat. No age, breed, or sex predilection exists. Pemphigus vegetans is believed to be a benign variant of pemphigus vulgaris.

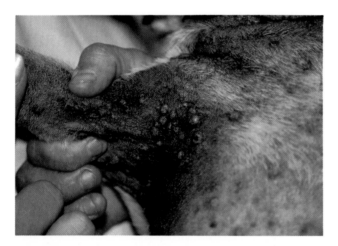

Figure 4-35   *Axillary area of 8-year-old Pug with pemphigus vegetans. Numerous firm, flat-topped pustules are evident.*

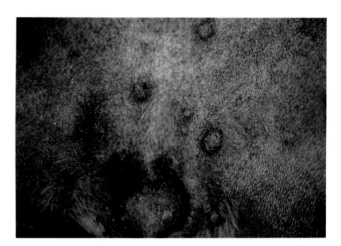

Figure 4-36   *Vulva and perivulvar area of Pug shown in Figure 4-35. Firm, flat-topped pustules in various stages of development are seen.*

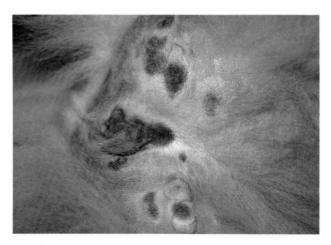

Figure 4-37   *Five-year-old Chow Chow with pemphigus vegetans. Vulvar and perivulvar areas show hyperpigmented patches containing pustules. (Red pen markings denote areas to be biopsied.)*

Canine Pemphigoid (Bullous Pemphigoid)

CLINICAL SIGNS

1. Ulcerations involve the oral cavity, mucocutaneous junctions, and/or skin
2. About 75% of patients have oral cavity involvement
3. The most common sites of skin lesions are the axillary and inguinal areas
4. Affected animals usually have pain
5. Patients are rarely pruritic
6. Most patients suffer from anorexia, depression, and/or weight loss

DIFFERENTIAL DIAGNOSIS

1. Pemphigus vulgaris
2. Systemic lupus erythematosus
3. Drug eruption
4. Toxic epidermal necrolysis
5. Lymphoreticular neoplasia

DIAGNOSTIC AIDS

1. Skin biopsies for histopathologic examination reveals subepidermal vacuolar alteration and vesicle formation
2. Biopsies for immunofluorescence usually positive
3. Indirect immunofluorescence is negative
4. Antinuclear antibody (ANA) test is negative

COMMENTS

Canine pemphigoid is a rare autoimmune skin disease of the dog. It has not been reported in the cat. There is no age or sex predilection. Collies and Shetland Sheepdogs may be predisposed. In the past bullous pemphigoid may have been misdiagnosed as hidradenitis suppurativa.

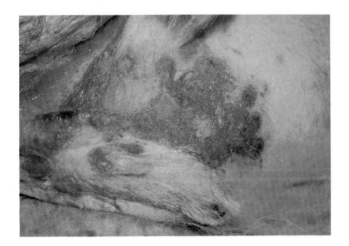

Figure 4-38 Ten-year-old Collie with pemphigoid. Extensive ulceration is seen in inguinal area. Lesions were quite painful. Patient was anorectic and febrile.

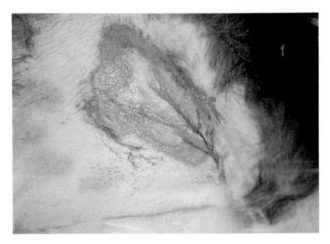

Figure 4-39 Left axillary area of Collie shown in Figure 4-38.

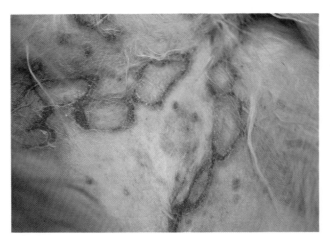

Figure 4-40 *Thirteen-year-old Shetland Sheepdog with canine pemphigoid. Note coalescing, serpiginous configuration of ulcerative lesions in inguinal area.*

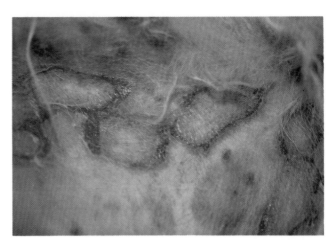

Figure 4-41 *Closer view of lesions shown in Figure 4-40.*

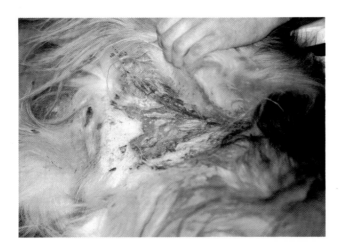

Figure 4-42 *Inguinal area of Collie with canine pemphigoid. Since bullae are very short-lived, most common presenting sign is extensive ulcerative lesions.*

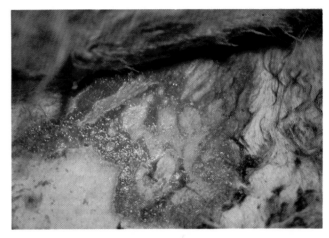

Figure 4-43 *Closer view of lesions in inguinal area of patient shown in Figure 4-42.*

Systemic Lupus Erythematosus

CLINICAL SIGNS

1. Skin lesions associated with this disease are quite diverse
2. Facial dermatitis is common and may assume a "butterfly" pattern
3. Mucocutaneous ulcerations are common
4. Seborrheic dermatoses
5. Glomerulonephritis, polyarthritis, anemia, lymphadenopathy, and fever may also be present

DIFFERENTIAL DIAGNOSIS

1. Pemphigus vulgaris
2. Discoid lupus erythematosus
3. Canine pemphigoid
4. Seborrheic skin disease
5. Demodicosis
6. Dermatophyte infection
7. Bacterial dermatitis
8. Toxic epidermal necrolysis
9. Lymphoreticular neoplasia

DIAGNOSTIC AIDS

1. Skin biopsies for histopathologic examination reveals lichenoid interface dermatitis or stomatitis and intraepidermal vesicular dermatitis
2. Biopsies for immunofluorescence are positive
3. Indirect immunofluorescence is negative
4. Lupus erythematosus cell test is negative
5. Antinuclear antibody (ANA) test is usually positive

COMMENTS

Systemic lupus erythematosus is a rare autoimmune disease with multisystemic signs. The skin and/or oral cavity is involved in about 30% of patients. The disease has been reported in the dog and cat. There is no known age or sex predilection. Collies, German Shepherd Dogs, Shetland Sheepdogs, and Siamese cats may be predisposed.

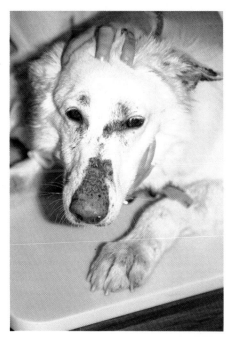

Figure 4-44 Six-year-old white German Shepherd Dog with systemic lupus erythematosus. Note hypopigmentation of nose and erythematous, ulcerative, crusted lesions on bridge of nose. Periocular areas are involved to lesser extent.

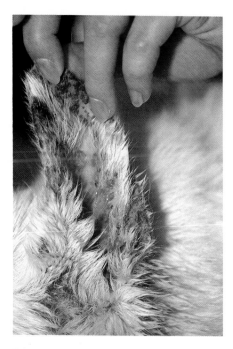

Figure 4-45 Severely ulcerated medial aspect of left ear pinna of patient shown in Figure 4-44.

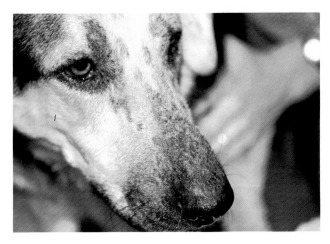

Figure 4-46   *Facial dermatitis in "butterfly" pattern on face of German Shepherd Dog with systemic lupus erythematosus. Note alopecia, erythema, erosions, pustules, and crusts.*

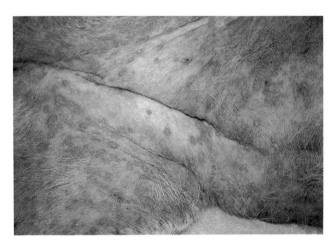

Figure 4-47   *Abdominal and inguinal areas of patient shown in Figure 4-46. Lesions are erythematous macules with pustules.*

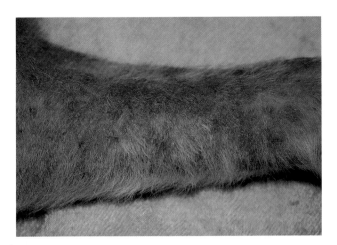

Figure 4-48   *Medial aspect of foreleg of lupus patient shown in Figures 4-46 and 4-47.*

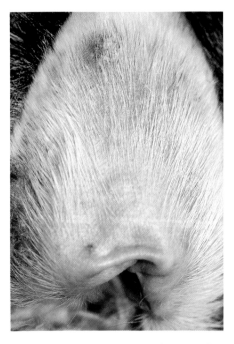

Figure 4-49   *Erythema, papules, pustules, and blisters on medial aspect of ear pinna of patient shown in Figures 4-46 to 4-48.*

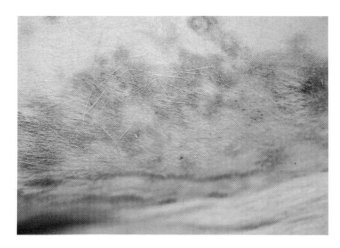

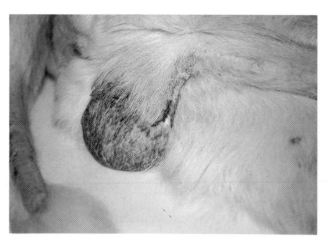

Figure 4-50   *Patchy erythema with some pustule and bullae formation on chest of mixed-breed dog with systemic lupus erythematosus.*

Figure 4-51   *Ulcerated scrotum of patient shown in Figure 4-50.*

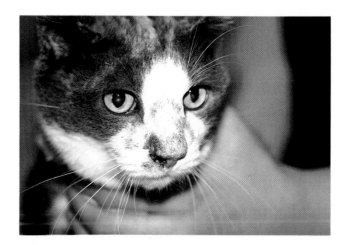

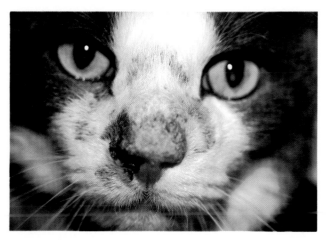

Figure 4-52   *Twelve-year-old Domestic Short-Haired cat shows facial lesions consisting of alopecia, erythema, and crusts. Ear pinnae and head are also involved.*

Figure 4-53   *Closer view of patient shown in Figure 4-52.*

Discoid Lupus Erythematosus

CLINICAL SIGNS

1. Lesions are most frequently found on the nose and bridge of nose. Other areas include the lips, periocular areas, ear pinnae, and distal limbs
2. Hypopigmentation, depigmentation, erythema, and scaling of the nose are often the earliest signs
3. Crusting, erosions, and ulcerations may develop

DIFFERENTIAL DIAGNOSIS

1. Pemphigus erythematosus
2. Pemphigus foliaceus
3. Systemic lupus erythematosus
4. Nasal pyoderma
5. Nasal solar dermatitis
6. Demodicosis
7. Dermatomyositis
8. Nasal hyperkeratosis

DIAGNOSTIC AIDS

1. Skin biopsies for histopathologic examination reveal hydropic and lichenoid interface dermatitis
2. Biopsies for direct immunofluorescence may be positive
3. Indirect immunofluorescence is negative
4. Antinuclear antibody (ANA) test is negative

COMMENTS

Discoid lupus erythematosus is the second most common form of autoimmune disease reported in the dog. (Pemphigus foliaceus is the most common.) It has not been reported in the cat. There is no age or sex predilection. Collies, Shetland Sheepdogs, German Shepherd Dogs, and Siberian Huskies may be predisposed. The lesions may be exacerbated by exposure to sunlight. Diseases that in the past were diagnosed as "nasal solar dermatosis" and "collie nose" may actually be discoid lupus erythematosus.

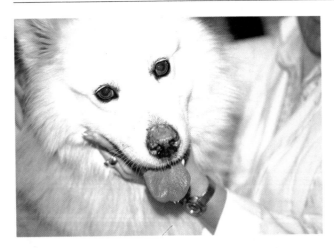

Figure 4-54 *Samoyed with discoid lupus erythematosus. Nose is depigmented, erythematous, and ulcerated.*

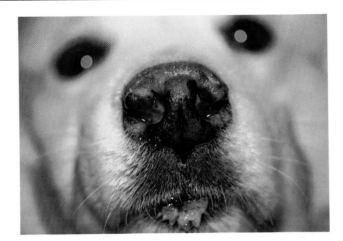

Figure 4-55 *Closer view of patient shown in Figure 4-54.*

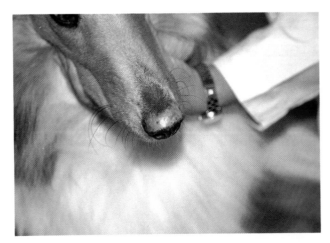

Figure 4-56 *Five-year-old Collie with depigmentation and erythema of nose.*

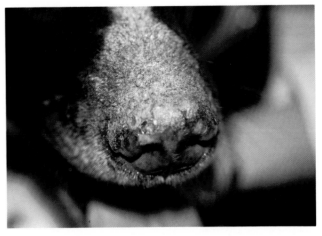

Figure 4-57 *Labrador Retriever with discoid lupus erythematosus. Nose is hypopigmented, with ulcers and crusts. Bridge of nose is severely crusted.*

Cold Agglutinin Disease

CLINICAL SIGNS

1. Lesions usually involve the extremities, tip of tail, ear pinnae, footpads, and/or nose
2. Lesions include ulceration, necrosis, erythema, and purpura
3. The lesions are caused or exacerbated by cold

DIFFERENTIAL DIAGNOSIS

1. Systemic lupus erythematosus
2. Frostbite
3. Vasculitis
4. Dermatomyositis

DIAGNOSTIC AIDS

1. In vitro autohemagglutination of blood at room temperature
2. Skin biopsies for histopathologic examination reveal necrosis and ulceration; some sections may demonstrate thrombosed-to-necrotic blood vessels
3. Biopsies for direct immunofluorescence may be positive
4. Coombs' test at 4° C is positive
5. Antinuclear antibody (ANA) test is negative

COMMENTS

Cold agglutinin disease is a rare autoimmune disease which has been reported in the dog and cat. No age, breed or sex predilection exists. The disease is associated with cold reacting erythrocyte autoantibodies, usually IgM, which are most active at 0° to 4° C. Cold agglutinin disease is a type II hypersensitivity reaction.

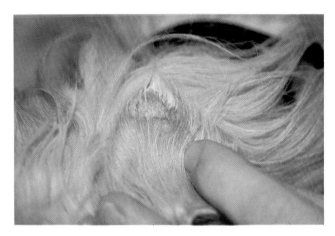

Figure 4-58　*Tip of ear pinna of 8-year-old Maltese. Note bluish hue of ear tip and erythematous border signifying vascular deficit. (Two weeks after this photograph was taken, ear tip fell off.)*

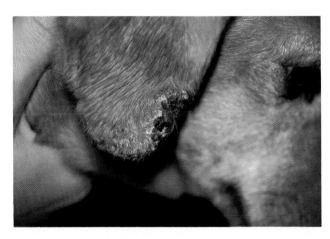

Figure 4-59　*Right ear pinna of 13-year-old Beagle. Entire ear pinna is edematous and ear pinnal tip is alopecic, erythematous, and necrotic.*

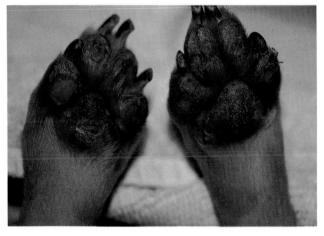

Figure 4-60　*Footpads of rear feet of patient shown in Figure 4-59 show central ulceration.*

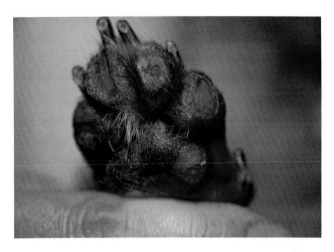

Figure 4-61　*Ulcerated footpads on forefoot of patient shown in Figures 4-59 and 4-60.*

PARASITIC DERMATOSES

Demodicosis (demodectic mange)

Sarcoptic mange

Notoedric mange (feline scabies)

Cheyletiella dermatitis

Otodectes cynotis (ear mites)

Tick bite dermatitis

Pelodera dermatitis (rhabditic dermatitis)

Hookworm dermatitis (ancylostomiasis, uncinariasis)

Heartworm dermatitis (dirofilariasis)

Pediculosis (louse infestation)

Demodicosis (Demodectic Mange)

CLINICAL SIGNS: LOCALIZED DEMODICOSIS

1. One to five areas on the body will show demodectic mites on skin scrapings
2. Involved areas are usually alopecic and erythemic, often with fine white scales or seborrheic dermatosis
3. A bacterial folliculitis may be clinically evident
4. Lesions are most common on the face (especially the periocular areas) head and feet
5. Pruritus is usually mild to absent

CLINICAL SIGNS: GENERALIZED DEMODICOSIS

1. More than five areas on the body will show demodectic mites on skin scrapings
2. Involved areas are usually alopecic and seborrheic
3. Secondary bacterial folliculitis and/or furunculosis are common
4. Pruritus is quite variable
5. Ceruminous otitis may be seen
6. Pododermatitis (which may be quite severe and painful) is frequently present
7. Severely involved animals may be febrile, anorectic, and lethargic

DIFFERENTIAL DIAGNOSIS

1. Bacterial dermatitis
2. Seborrheic dermatitis
3. Dermatophyte infection
4. Canine acne
5. Juvenile pyoderma
6. Pemphigus foliaceus and pemphigus vulgaris
7. Dermatomyositis
8. Lupus erythematosus

DIAGNOSTIC AIDS

1. Skin scrapings are diagnostic
2. Biopsies for histopathologic examination are also diagnostic, but rarely necessary
3. Mites are occasionally found in fecal floatations, however, this simply indicates that the patient has ingested mites while licking or biting involved areas of the skin

COMMENTS

Juvenile demodicosis usually occurs in dogs between the ages of 4 and 18 months. Certain breeds of dogs are predisposed. These include Doberman Pinschers, Boxers, Great Danes, Collies, Chow Chows, and Short-Haired Dachshunds. Generalized juvenile-onset demodicosis is hereditary, and affected canines should not be used in breeding programs. Localized juvenile-onset demodicosis is not considered to be hereditary. Adult-onset demodicosis may occur at any age and may be associated with internal diseases and neoplasia. Demodicosis is rare in the cat.

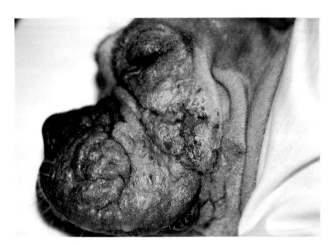

Figure 5-1 *Nine-month-old Boxer has facial alopecia with areas of hyperpigmentation and erythema. Pustular dermatitis and areas of excoriation are also evident.*

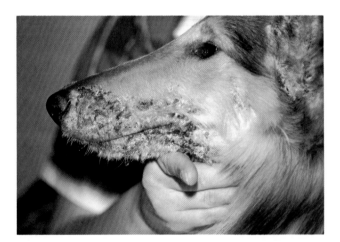

Figure 5-2 *Alopecia, erythema, and crusting on muzzle, cheek, and preauricular area of 6-month-old Collie. Patient's generalized demodicosis was mildly pruritic.*

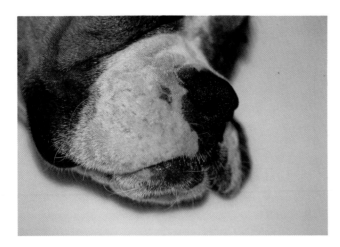

Figure 5-3 *Mild alopecia and erythema on muzzle of 10-month-old Boxer. No other clinical signs were associated with this patient's localized demodicosis.*

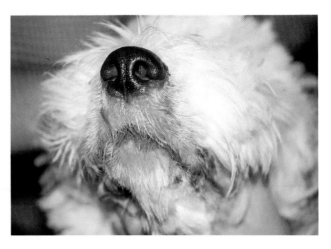

Figure 5-4 *Twelve-year-old Old English Sheepdog with muzzle erythema and alopecia. Patient also had severe pododermatitis and truncal lesions associated with his generalized demodicosis.*

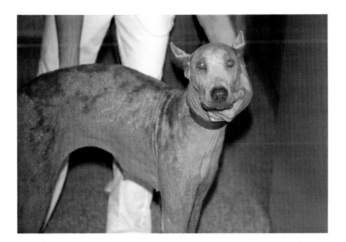

Figure 5-5 *"Blue"-colored Doberman Pinscher youngster with near-total alopecia and scaling.*

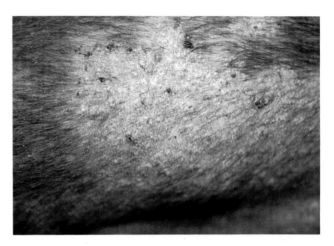

Figure 5-6 *Closer view of patient shown in Figure 5-5. Note marked scaling and pustules, some with hemorrhagic crusts.*

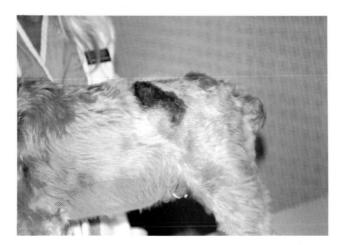

Figure 5-7 *Patch of alopecia and hyperpigmentation on trunk of 7-year-old Miniature Schnauzer with localized demodicosis.*

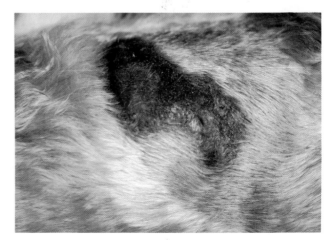

Figure 5-8 *Closer view of lesion shown in previous photograph. In addition to obvious alopecia and hyperpigmentation, there is some scaling and pustule formation. Cause of patient's adult-onset demodicosis was not detected.*

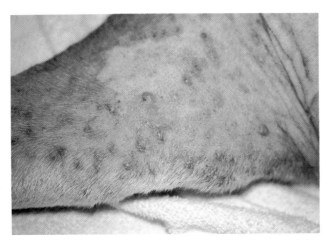

Figure 5-9 *Medial thigh of 13-month-old Pit Bull Terrier. Note numerous pustules and alopecia. More than 50 demodectic mites were found per skin scraping.*

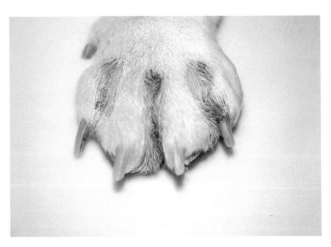

Figure 5-10 *Left forefoot of patient shown in Figure 5-9. Interdigital erythema and swelling are seen. Patient had pedal pruritus with occasional limping.*

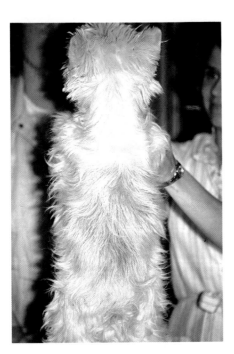

Figure 5-11 *Back of 11-month-old West Highland White Terrier. Thinned haircoat and seborrhea oleosa is evident. Many demodectic mites were found on skin scrapings. No other areas were involved.*

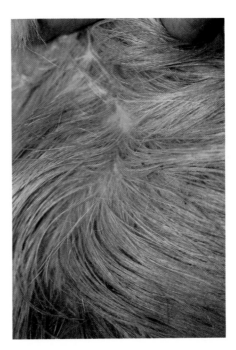

Figure 5-12 *Closer view of seborrhea oleosa shown in Figure 5-11. Patient was moderately pruritic.*

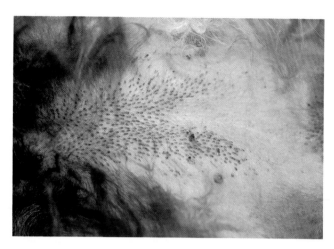

Figure 5-13 *Follicular plugging (comedone or blackhead formation) in inguinal area of mature Lhasa Apso. Hundreds of demodectic mites were found in scrapings taken from this area.*

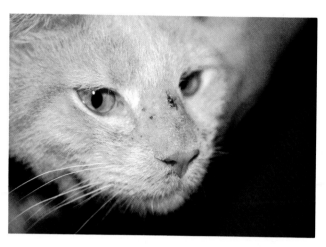

Figure 5-14 *Alopecia, erythema, and excoriation on face of 6-year-old Domestic Short-Haired cat. Demodectic mites were not found on other areas of body.*

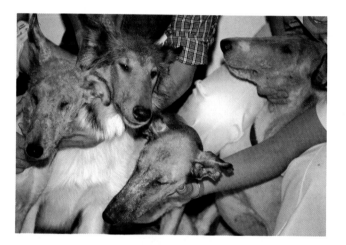

Figure 5-15 *Litter of 5-month-old Collie pups demonstrate that juvenile-onset generalized demodicosis is hereditary.*

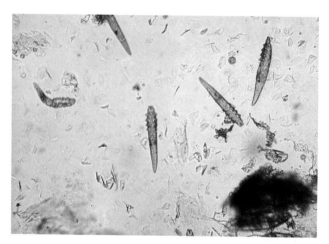

Figure 5-16 *Mineral oil preparation of* Demodex canis *(×100). Adult mites (four pairs of legs) and skin debris are seen.*

Sarcoptic Mange

CLINICAL SIGNS

1. Intense pruritus is the hallmark of sarcoptic mange
2. Areas most frequently involved are the ear pinnal margins, elbows, hocks, and abdomen; however, any and all areas of the body may be involved
3. Self-induced alpecia, scaling, crusting, and bloody excoriations are common
4. Hyperpigmentation, lichenification, and/or seborrheic skin disease may be the result of constant pruritus
5. Patients are often pruritic in the examination room and owners often report that patients are awake and scratching during the night

DIFFERENTIAL DIAGNOSIS

1. Allergic inhalant disease (atopy)
2. Food hypersensitivity
3. Contact dermatitis
4. Cheyletiella infestation
5. Bacterial folliculitis
6. Dermatophyte infection
7. Seborrheic dermatitis
8. Pediculosis

DIAGNOSTIC AIDS

1. Sarcoptic mites (unlike demodectic mites) may be very difficult to find on skin scrapings. The author has had greatest success in finding mites on scrapings taken from the ear pinnal margins
2. Response to treatment is a very important diagnostic aid when skin scrapings are negative

COMMENTS

Canine sarcoptic mange is considered to be highly contagious; however, the author has seen numerous cases where contact household dogs did not develop clinical signs, even after 6 months of exposure to a scabetic canine. Therefore involvement of other dogs in the home should not be a diagnostic factor. Canine sarcoptic mites are capable of burrowing in human skin, laying eggs, and producing an intensely pruritic transient dermatitis. The mites survive in household environments for short periods of time. The most common routes of transmission are via direct contact with scabetic canines and contaminated grooming instruments.

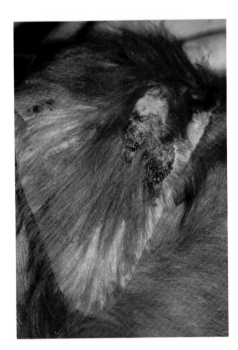

Figure 5-17 Ear pinna of Golden Retriever with sarcoptic mange. Note significant self-induced alopecia, crusting along pinnal margins, and excoriations.

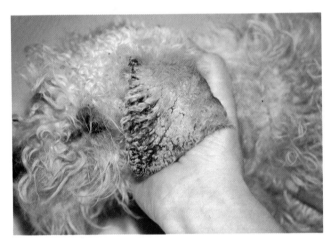

Figure 5-18 Thick crusts and fissures are seen on ear pinna of this 6-month-old Bichon Frise with sarcoptic mange. Hundreds of mites were found on scrapings taken from ear pinnae.

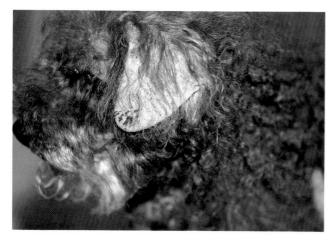

Figure 5-19   *Ear pinna of 8-year-old Poodle with sarcoptic mange. Note self-induced alopecia with some crust formation. Apparently dog became infested at grooming parlor by "contaminated" clipper blades.*

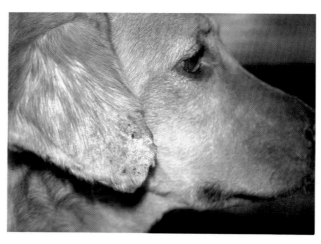

Figure 5-20   *Mixed-breed dog shows ear pinnal alopecia, erythema, and excoriated papules. Patient also had excoriations on elbows and abdomen.*

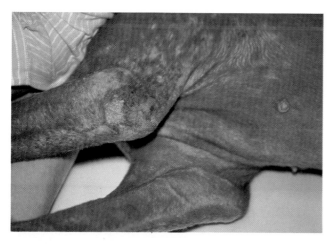

Figure 5-21   *Excoriated elbow and axillary areas of 7-year-old Weimaraner with sarcoptic mange. Skin scrapings from crusted area on elbow were positive for* Sarcoptes scabiei.

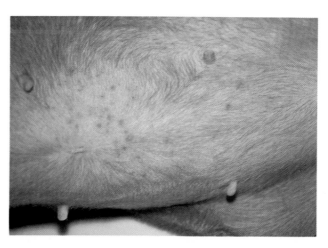

Figure 5-22   *Abdomen of patient shown in Figure 5-21. Intensely pruritic abdominal rash is common finding in scabetic patients.*

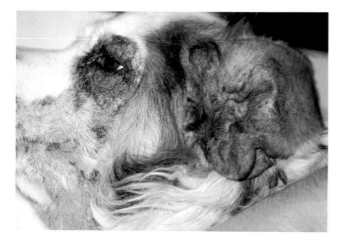

Figure 5-23   *Eleven-year-old mixed-breed dog with 2-year history of severe generalized pruritus. Note periocular alopecia and hyperpigmentation and muzzle erythema. Otitis externa was secondary to chronic pruritus and inflammation.*

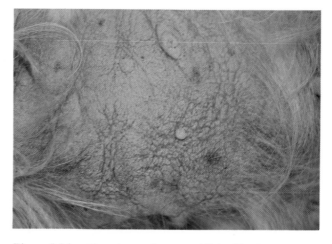

Figure 5-24   *Alopecia, erythema, and lichenification on abdomen of patient shown in Figure 5-23. Patient's sarcoptic mange had been misdiagnosed as allergies.*

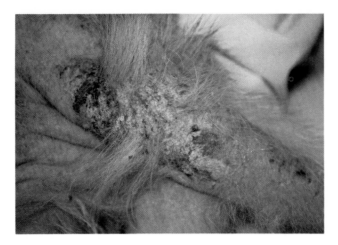

Figure 5-25   *Severely crusted elbow of scabetic Keeshond. Patient also had generalized near-total self-induced alopecia and erythema.*

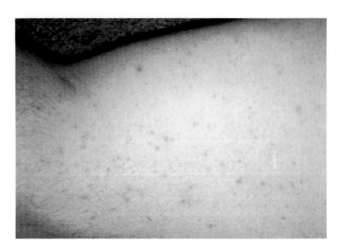

Figure 5-26   *Pruritic rash on arm of owner of Keeshond shown in Figure 5-25. Intensely pruritic, usually transient, dermatitis may be seen in humans who have contact with scabetic canines.*

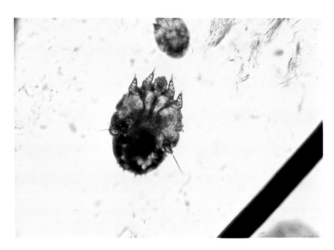

Figure 5-27   *Skin scraping in mineral oil shows gravid female* Sarcoptes scabiei var. canis *mite. (×100).*

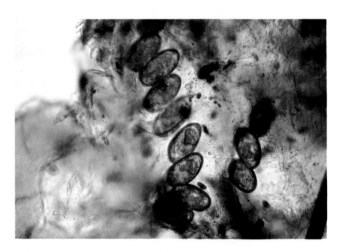

Figure 5-28   *Skin scraping shows numerous* Sarcoptes scabiei *eggs and skin debris. (×100).*

Notoedric Mange (Feline Scabies)

CLINICAL SIGNS

1. Lesions are most common on the head, neck, and ear pinnae
2. Other areas of frequent involvement include the feet and abdomen; however, any part of the body may be involved
3. Intense pruritus results in self-induced alopecia, erythema, and excoriations
4. Papules and crusts may also be seen

DIFFERENTIAL DIAGNOSIS

1. *Otodectes cynotis* (ear mites)
2. Cheyletiella dermatitis
3. Dermatophyte infection
4. Food hypersensitivity
5. Allergic inhalant disease
6. Flea bite hypersensitivity
7. Pemphigus foliaceus

DIAGNOSTIC AIDS

1. Mites are usually quite easy to find on skin scrapings. The mites are similar in appearance to canine scabies mites but they are smaller
2. In some cases in which mites cannot be demonstrated, response to miticidal treatment may be the only way to make a definitive diagnosis

COMMENTS

Notoedric mange should always be considered in patients presented for head and neck pruritus. Contact cats are frequently involved; however, as with canine scabies, a diagnosis of notoedric mange should not be ruled out if contact cats are not involved. The mites may cause a transient pruritic dermatitis in contact humans and dogs, but the mites are incapable of completing their life cycles on these species.

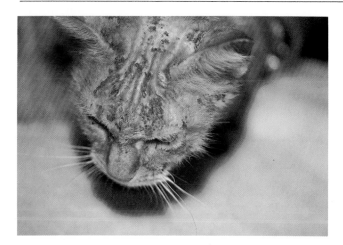

Figure 5-29 Face and head of 3-year-old Domestic Short-Haired cat with notoedric mange. Self-induced alopecia and excoriated papules are evident.

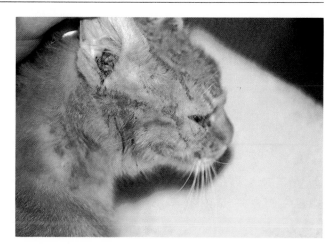

Figure 5-30 Excoriations on right side of face of patient shown in Figure 5-29. Intense pruritus is hallmark of this disease.

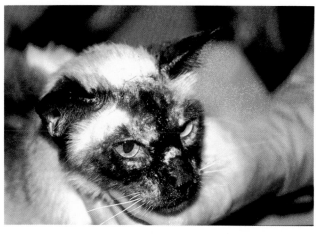

Figure 5-31 Alopecia, scaling, and crusting on face and ears of young Siamese cat with notoedric mange.

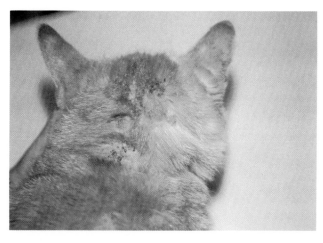

Figure 5-32 Self-induced alopecia, erythema, and some excoriations on neck and ears of cat with notoedric mange.

Cheyletiella Dermatitis

CLINICAL SIGNS

1. The most common sign is mild scaling which looks like seborrhea sicca
2. Pruritus varies from intense to moderate to absent
3. Patients may be totally asymptomatic

DIFFERENTIAL DIAGNOSIS

1. The numerous other causes of seborrhea sicca
2. Other mite infestations such as *Sarcoptes scabiei, Notoedres cati,* and *Otodectes cynotis* (These diseases are usually much more pruritic than cheyletiella dermatitis.)

DIAGNOSTIC AIDS

1. Mites are sometimes seen walking on the hair surface either with the naked eye or using a magnifying loop. Hence term "walking dandruff"
2. Comb preparations using a flea comb, and then examining the scale and seborrheic debris under microscope is helpful
3. Cellophane tape may be used to gather skin scale. The tape is then applied to a microscope slide and examined

COMMENTS

The most common cheyletiella mites affecting dogs and cats are *C. yasguri, C. parasitovorax,* and *C. blakei.* Young animals are most frequently affected. The mites are not host specific and may live in the environment for several days. The mites are capable of causing an intensely pruritic, transient dermatitis in human contacts.

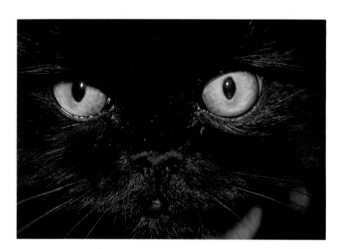

Figure 5-33 *White specks on face of this young Persian cat are Cheyletiella mites. Patient was mildly pruritic and showed no other clinical signs.*

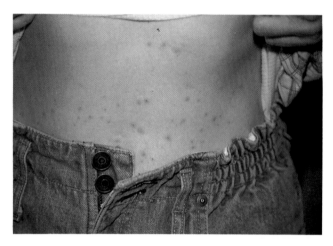

Figure 5-34 *Abdomen of owner of cat with Cheyletiella dermatitis. This human contact had intensely pruritic papular eruption over most of her trunk.*

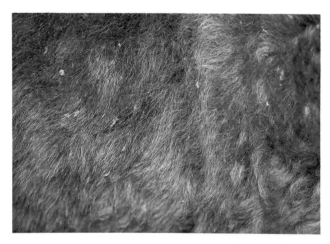

Figure 5-35 *Miniature Schnauzer with seborrheic flakes that contained Cheyletiella mites. Patient was presented for his "dandruff" and was not pruritic.*

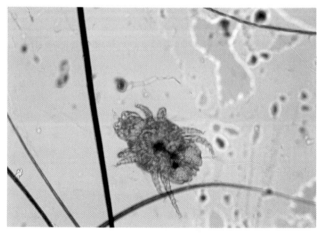

Figure 5-36 *Mineral oil preparation shows adult Cheyletiella mite. (×100).*

Otodectes cynotis (Ear Mites)

CLINICAL SIGNS

1. The hallmark of *Otodectes cynotis* infestation is otitis externa which is manifested by a black, brown, or reddish brown exudate in the external ear canal
2. Pruritus is moderate to severe
3. Mites and lesions may also be found on the head, neck, rump, and tail

DIFFERENTIAL DIAGNOSIS

1. Notoedric mange (cats)
2. Sarcoptic mange (dogs)
3. Food hypersensitivity
4. Allergic inhalant disease
5. Flea bite hypersensitivity

DIAGNOSTIC AIDS

1. It is very important to demonstrate the mites in samples of crusts and cerumen taken from the external ear canal. Other diseases are often misdiagnosed as *Otodectes cynotis* simply because large amounts of a dark ear discharge is present
2. Mites have uncommonly been found on skin scrapings taken from the head, neck and rump

COMMENTS

Otodectes cynotis is a common cause of head and neck pruritus in dogs and cats. It is an infrequent cause of truncal pruritus. The mites are not host specific. Successful treatment involves not only treatment of the external ear canals but also the use of an insecticide on the trunk.

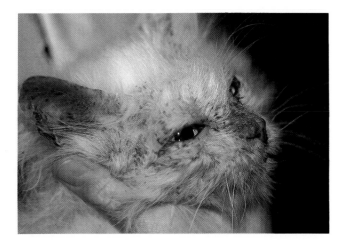

Figure 5-37 *Self-induced alopecia with papules and crusts on face and ears of patient with ear mites.*

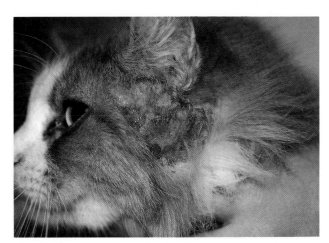

Figure 5-38 *Bloody excoriation on face of young cat. Patient's intense pruritus was caused by* Otodectes cynotis.

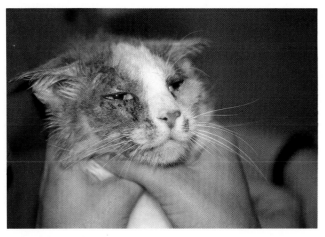

Figure 5-39 *Domestic Short-Haired cat with numerous facial excoriations. Lesions and "ear" mites were also present on rump and tail; this emphasizes need for total body treatment.*

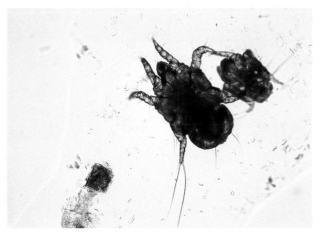

Figure 5-40 Otodectes cynotis *mites in mineral oil preparation from external ear canal of patient shown in Figure 5-39. (×100).*

Tick Bite Dermatitis

CLINICAL SIGNS

1. The most common sign is an erythematous papule at the site of tick attachment
2. Occasionally patients show hypersensitivity reactions
3. Most patients are not pruritic
4. Tick-borne diseases may result in a myriad of clinical signs
5. A foreign body granuloma may develop at the site of tick attachment, especially if only part of the tick is removed

DIFFERENTIAL DIAGNOSIS

There are virtually no differential diagnoses since ticks are easy to find and identify.

DIAGNOSTIC AIDS

A thorough physical examination is diagnostic since ticks are usually quite apparent and identifiable.

COMMENTS

Ticks are not considered to be host specific. They are capable of surviving in the environment for several months or longer. Although ticks are capable of producing a hypersensitivity reaction in their hosts, the major problems associated with tick infestation are the diseases they are capable of spreading. These include bacterial, rickettsial, viral, and protozoan diseases.

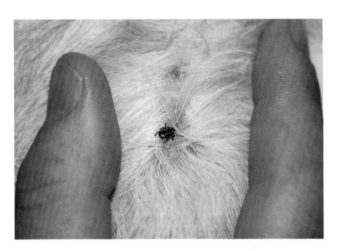

Figure 5-41 *Tick attached to epidermis on lateral thoracic area of mixed-breed dog. Note papule above tick which is site of previous tick attachment.*

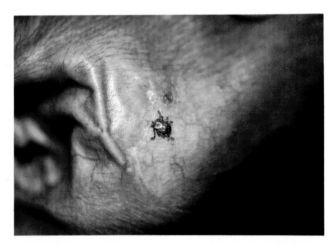

Figure 5-42 *"American dog tick," Dermacentor variabilis, attached to medial aspect of ear pinna. This tick is capable of transmitting Rocky Mountain Spotted Tick Fever.*

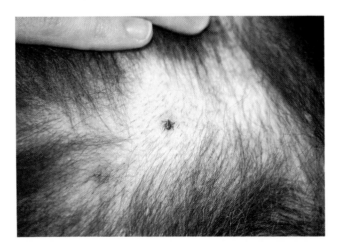

Figure 5-43 *Another "dog tick" attached to ventral chest area. Note erythema around site of tick attachment as well as previous tick bite below and to left of tick.*

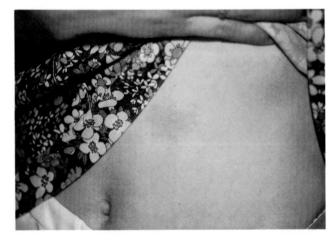

Figure 5-44 *Tick bite on abdomen of veterinary technician. Note marked peripheral erythema.*

Pelodera Dermatitis (Rhabditic Dermatitis)

CLINICAL SIGNS

1. Lesions are typically located on areas of the skin that contact the ground such as the feet, legs, perineum, and ventral chest
2. Involved areas are alopecic and erythematous
3. Chronic pruritus may lead to hyperpigmentation and lichenification
4. Pruritus is usually fairly intense and nonseasonal

DIFFERENTIAL DIAGNOSIS

1. Demodicosis
2. Sarcoptic mange
3. Hookworm dermatitis
4. Heartworm dermatitis
5. Allergic inhalant disease
6. Food hypersensitivity

DIAGNOSTIC AIDS

1. Skin scrapings reveal small, motile nematode larvae
2. History of poor sanitation and wet bedding in addition to contact with hay, straw, or rice hulls

COMMENTS

Pelodera dermatitis is an uncommon skin disease of dogs. It has not been reported in cats. The causative organism is a free-living nematode, *Pelodera strongyloides*. The larvae are incapable of penetrating normal skin. The skin must first be inflamed or macerated by constant damp environments.

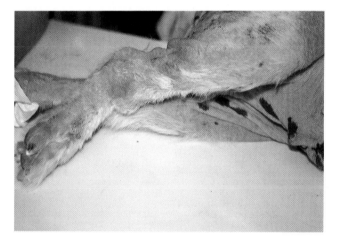

Figure 5-45   Rear legs and abdomen of 2-year-old hunting dog show marked self-induced alopecia and erythema. Patient was quite pruritic.

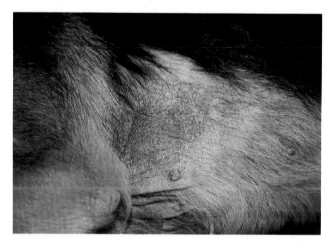

Figure 5-46   Constant pruritus of chest, elbows, and lateral thoracic area caused by Pelodera strongyloides *resulted in this patient's alopecia, with hyperpigmentation and peripheral erythema.*

Hookworm Dermatitis (Ancylostomiasis, Uncinariasis)

CLINICAL SIGNS

1. Areas most frequently involved include the feet, sternum, and bony prominences of the elbows and hocks. Other areas include the abdomen, legs, perineum, and perianal areas
2. The initial lesions are red papules that soon become erythematous patches
3. Involved skin is usually alopecic and erythemic.
4. Lichenification and hyperpigmentation may be seen in chronic cases
5. Patients are usually mildly to moderately pruritic

DIFFERENTIAL DIAGNOSIS

1. Demodicosis
2. Pelodera dermatitis
3. Allergic inhalant disease
4. Food hypersensitivity
5. Allergic contact dermatitis
6. Sarcoptic mange

DIAGNOSTIC AIDS

1. Finding hookworm eggs on fecal flotation
2. History of housing in dirt or grass runs or poor sanitation
3. Biopsies for histopathologic examination are often helpful but usually not diagnostic

COMMENTS

In most parts of the country hookworm dermatitis is an uncommon cause of pedal dermatitis and dermatitis involving "contact" areas of the skin. The disease is caused by larvae of *Ancylostoma caninum, Ancylostoma braziliense,* or *Uncinaria stenocephala.* Hookworm dermatitis must be considered, when the patient is housed in earth or grass runs and when the areas of involvement are the feet or contact areas. Finding hookworm eggs on fecal flotation does *not* make a definitive diagnosis since the hookworms may be an incidental finding or they may simply be a complicating factor in any of the differential diagnoses.

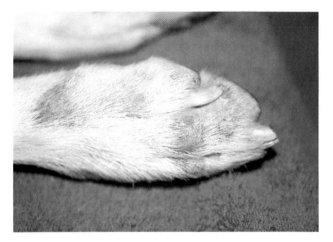

Figure 5-47 *Areas of self-induced alopecia and erythema on forefoot of young dog with hookworm dermatitis.*

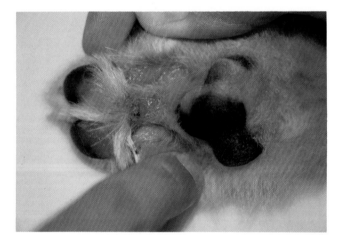

Figure 5-48 *Interdigital spaces on forefoot of 4-year-old mixed-breed dog with* Ancylostoma caninum. *Note significant erythema and some areas of ulceration.*

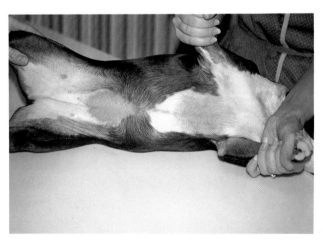

Figure 5-49 *Erythematous patches on ventrum of young Boston Terrier. Patient was moderately pruritic.*

Heartworm Dermatitis (Dirofilariasis)

CLINICAL SIGNS

1. Multiple ulcerated nodules or plaques
2. Lesions are usually alopecic
3. Areas of involvement include the head, ventral trunk and proximal extremities
4. Patients are usually very pruritic

DIFFERENTIAL DIAGNOSIS

1. Bacterial dermatitis
2. Dermatophyte infection
3. Neoplasia
4. Sporotrichosis

DIAGNOSTIC AIDS

1. Finding microfilaria of *Dirofilaria immitis* in blood samples
2. Skin biopsies for histopathologic examination reveal pyogranulomatous dermatitis and microfilarial segments within the granulomas
3. Skin scrapings are not diagnostic

COMMENTS

Heartworm dermatitis is an uncommon cause of nodular, ulcerative, pruritic dermatitis in the dog. No age, breed, or sex predilection has been reported. Finding microfilaria of *Dirofilaria immitis* in blood samples does *not* make a definitive diagnosis of heartworm dermatitis, since the microfilaria may be an incidental finding or they may be a complicating factor and not the sole cause of the patient's dermatitis.

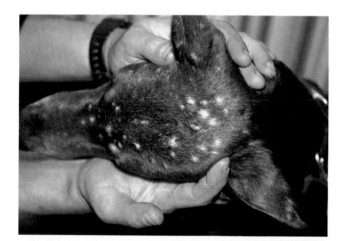

Figure 5-50   *Alopecic, nodular lesions with some ulceration on head of young Doberman Pinscher with heartworm dermatitis.*

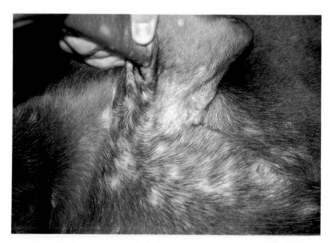

Figure 5-51   *Axillary area of Doberman shown in Figure 5-50. Extensive alopecic, erythemic nodules are seen. Patient was quite pruritic.*

Pediculosis (Louse Infestation)

CLINICAL SIGNS

1. The most common sign in the dog is mild, generalized seborrhea sicca
2. The most common sign in the cat is miliary dermatitis
3. Pruritus varies from nonexistent to fairly severe
4. Pruritic patients have varying degrees of self-induced alopecia and excoriations
5. Dogs and cats may be asymptomatic carriers

DIFFERENTIAL DIAGNOSIS

1. Seborrheic dermatitis
2. Cheyletiella dermatitis
3. Dermatophyte infection
4. Allergic dermatitis (flea, food, inhalant)
5. Sarcoptic or notoedric mange

DIAGNOSTIC AIDS

1. Physical examination usually reveals the lice. A magnifying lens or loop is helpful
2. The cellophane tape technique is helpful. Press the tape against skin scale and debris on the patient's skin. Then apply the tape to a slide and examine under a microscope for lice and eggs.

COMMENTS

Pediculosis is an uncommon cause of dermatitis in most veterinary practices. Lice are easily killed by most flea products, including shampoos and powders. Therefore pediculosis is usually a disease of filth and poor sanitation. Lice are host specific and spend their complete life cycles on the host. They are capable of living in the environment for only a few days.

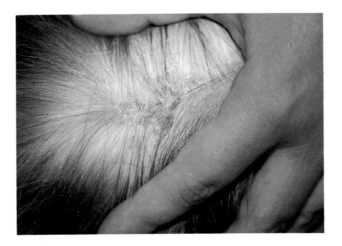

Figure 5-52   *Miliary dermatitis on midback of long-haired cat. Close examination reveals lice attached to hairs. This patient was moderately pruritic.*

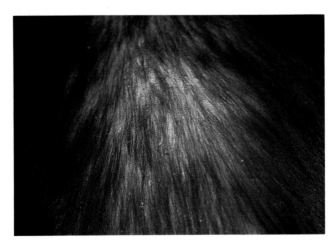

Figure 5-53   *Mild seborrheic dermatitis and alopecia on back of Irish Setter with pediculosis.*

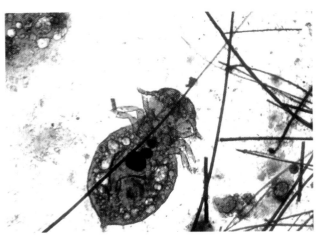

Figure 5-54   *Adult* Trichodectes canis, *the biting louse of dogs, found on skin scrapings from infested canine.*

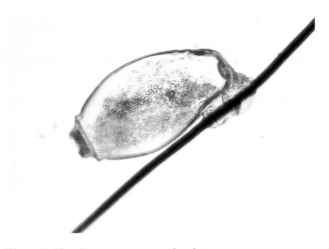

Figure 5-55   *Louse egg cemented to hair.*

ENDOCRINE DERMATOSES

Hyperadrenocorticism (Cushing's syndrome)

Adult-onset hyposomatotropism (adult-onset growth hormone deficiency, growth hormone–responsive alopecia)

Sertoli's cell tumor dermatopathy

Male feminizing syndrome

Testosterone-responsive dermatosis of male and female dogs

Ovarian imbalance (hyperestrogenism in female dogs)

Estrogen-responsive dermatosis of male and female dogs

Canine hypothyroidism

Feline hypothyroidism

Feline hyperthyroidism

Canine hypoadrenocorticism (Addison's disease)

Hyperadrenocorticism (Cushing's Syndrome)

CLINICAL SIGNS

1. Bilaterally symmetric truncal alopecia (The head and limbs are spared in most cases)
2. Some patients have easy epilation of truncal hair
3. Abnormalities of skin pigment (hypopigmentation or hyperpigmentation) in involved areas are common
4. Thin, hypotonic skin
5. Increased predisposition to bacterial skin infections
6. Poor wound healing
7. Prominent abdominal vasculature
8. Easy bruising
9. Seborrheic dermatoses
10. Comedone formation (follicular plugging)
11. Pruritus is rare
12. Calcinosis cutis
13. Pot-bellied appearance
14. Polydipsia, polyuria, and/or polyphagia
15. Muscle wasting

DIFFERENTIAL DIAGNOSIS

1. Hypothyroidism
2. Adult-onset hyposomatotropism
3. Sex hormone imbalances
4. Other diseases associated with polyuria and polydipsia such as diabetes mellitus and renal disease

DIAGNOSTIC AIDS

1. Complete blood count usually shows leukocytosis, neutrophilia, lymphopenia, and eosinopenia
2. Chemistry profile often shows elevated serum alkaline phosphatase
3. Adrenocorticotropic hormone (ACTH) stimulation tests
4. Dexamethasone (high and low dose) suppression tests
5. Most patients have a lowered total thyroxine level

COMMENTS

Hyperadrenocorticism may be naturally occurring due to an adrenal tumor, pituitary tumor, or adrenal hyperplasia. Breeds predisposed to develop naturally occurring hyperadrenocorticism include Miniature Poodles, Short-Haired Dachshunds, Boxers, and Boston Terriers. The disease may also be produced by the use of exogenous glucocorticoids in the treatment of pruritic skin diseases and other diseases.

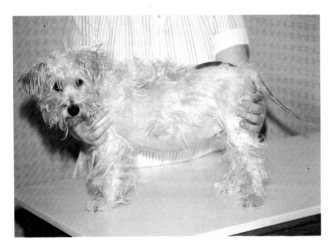

Figure 6-1   *Thirteen-year-old mixed-breed dog with alopecia of trunk and tail. Patient also has "pot-bellied" appearance.*

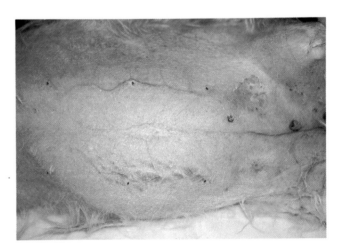

Figure 6-2   *Abdomen of patient shown in Figure 6-1. Note "pot-bellied" appearance, prominent abdominal vasculature, striae, and bacterial dermatitis.*

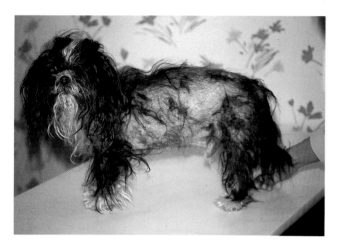

Figure 6-3   Ten-year-old Lhasa Apso with patchy truncal alopecia.

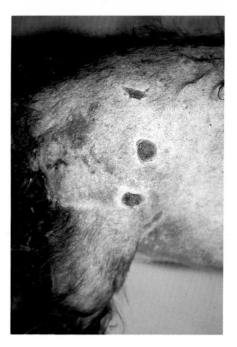

Figure 6-4   Right thigh of patient shown in Figure 6-3. Note alopecia and poor wound healing.

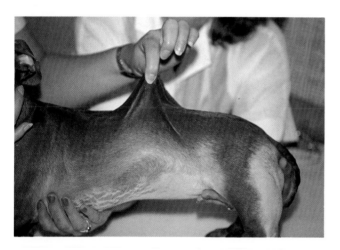

Figure 6-5   Four-year-old Short-Haired Dachshund with iatrogenic hyperadrenocorticism. Note hypotonic skin.

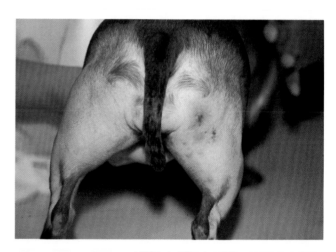

Figure 6-6   Alopecic caudal thighs of patient shown in Figure 6-5. Bacterial lesions are also evident.

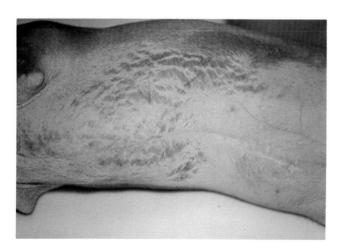

Figure 6-7   Ventral chest of patient in Figures 6-5 and 6-6. Striae and prominent abdominal vasculature are seen.

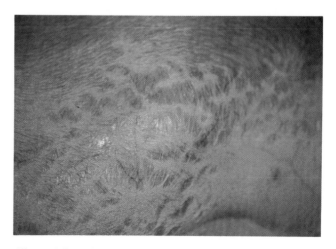

Figure 6-8   Closer view of striae shown in Figure 6-7.

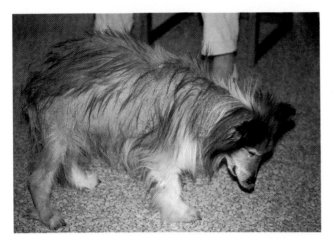

Figure 6-9   *Twelve-year-old Shetland Sheepdog with advanced hyperadrenocorticism. Patient has marked truncal alopecia. Widebased stance is indicative of muscle weakness.*

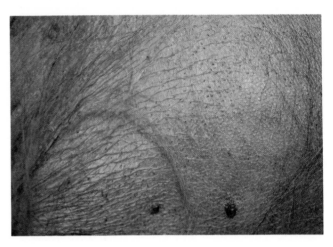

Figure 6-10   *Closer view of Sheltie shown in Figure 6-9. Note very thin skin and follicular plugging.*

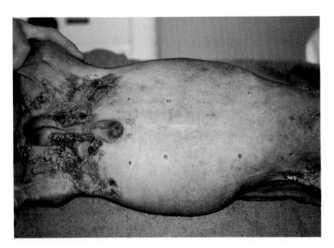

Figure 6-11   *Abdominal and inguinal areas of 7-year-old Short-Haired Dachshund. Note "pot-bellied" appearance, prominent abdominal vasculature, and extensive calcinosus cutis.*

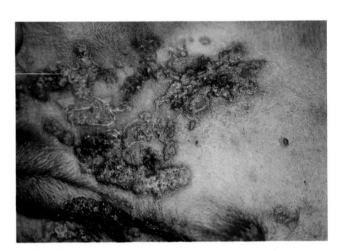

Figure 6-12   *Closer view of calcinosus cutis lesions shown in Figure 6-11.*

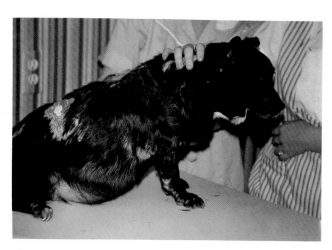

Figure 6-13   *Mixed-breed dog with adrenal hyperplasia. Note "pot-bellied" appearance, patchy truncal alopecia, and area of calcinosus cutis.*

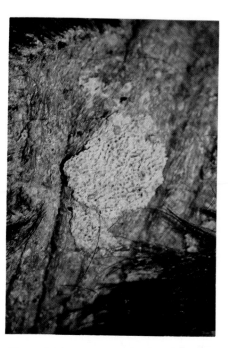

Figure 6-14   *Close-up photograph of calcium plaque on skin surface of patient shown in Figure 6-13.*

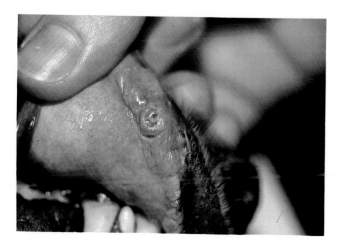

Figure 6-15   *Calcium deposits in lip of patient shown in Figures 6-13 and 6-14.*

Adult-Onset Hyposomatotropism (Adult-Onset Growth Hormone Deficiency, Growth Hormone–Responsive Alopecia)

CLINICAL SIGNS

1. Bilaterally symmetric alopecia of neck, trunk, tail and/or caudal thighs
2. Remaining truncal hair often has a "cotton candy" texture and appearance.
3. Skin in involved areas usually becomes hyperpigmented
4. Patients are not pruritic
5. Other than these cutaneous abnormalities, patients are healthy

DIFFERENTIAL DIAGNOSIS

1. Hyperadrenocorticism
2. Hypothyroidism
3. Sex hormone imbalances

DIAGNOSTIC AIDS

1. Rule out other endocrine alopecias
2. Skin biopsies for histopathologic examination may reveal decreased dermal elastin
3. Xylazine stimulation tests
4. Response to treatment with somatotropin

COMMENTS

Adult-onset hyposomatotropism is an uncommon disease of the dog. It has not been reported in the cat. Increased incidence of the disease has been reported in the Chow Chow, Pomeranian, Keeshond, and Miniature Poodle. Male dogs appear to be predisposed.

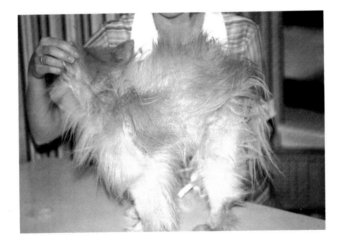

Figure 6-16 *Lateral view of 7-year-old Pomeranian shows alopecia of neck and trunk, with some hyperpigmentation.*

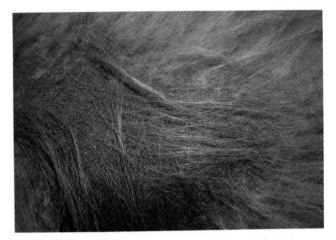

Figure 6-17 *Closer view of alopecic, hyperpigmented skin of Pomeranian shown in Figure 6-16.*

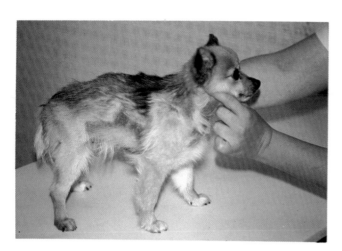

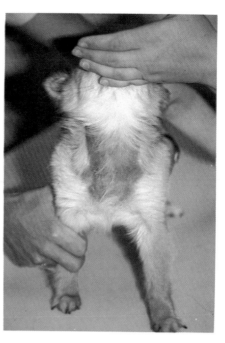

Figure 6-18   *Mixed Chihuahua with hyposomatotropism has alopecic, hyperpigmented skin.*

Figure 6-19   *Ventral neck of patient shown in Figure 6-18.*

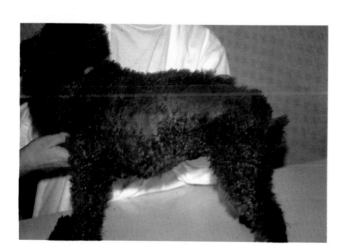

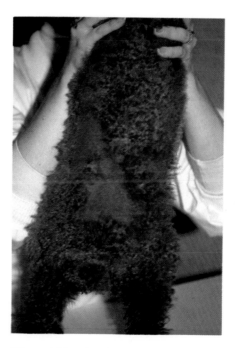

Figure 6-20   *Miniature Poodle with nonpruritic truncal alopecia and hyperpigmentation.*

Figure 6-21   *Another view of Poodle with adult-onset growth hormone deficiency shown in Figure 6-20.*

Sertoli's Cell Tumor Dermatopathy

CLINICAL SIGNS

1. Bilaterally symmetric alopecia usually involving the trunk, neck, abdomen, ventral chest, and/or thighs
2. Skin in involved areas may be hyperpigmented or show splotchy pigmentation called melanosis
3. Patients are rarely pruritic
4. Gynecomastia may be present
5. Pendulous prepuce
6. A line of erythema may extend from the scrotum to the tip of the prepuce
7. Patient may sexually attract other male dogs
8. Estrogen-induced bone marrow suppression (thrombocytopenia, neutropenia, anemia) has been reported

DIFFERENTIAL DIAGNOSIS

1. Hypothyroidism
2. Hyperadrenocorticism
3. Testosterone-responsive dermatosis
4. Male feminizing syndrome
5. Adult-onset hyposomatotropism

DIAGNOSTIC AIDS

1. Careful physical examination
2. Rule out other endocrine imbalances
3. Skin biopsies for histopathologic examination are not diagnostic
4. Blood estrogen levels may be helpful
5. Castration and histopathologic examination of testes

COMMENTS

The cutaneous changes in Sertoli's cell tumor dermatopathy are caused by estrogen secretion by neoplastic testicular cells. Functional Sertoli's cell tumors are found most commonly in retained testicles. Palpable Sertoli's cell tumors have also been found in scrotal testicles. Also, scrotal testicles that are normal on palpation may contain functional Sertoli's cell tumors. Middle-aged to older dogs are predisposed. Breed predilections are controversial. The disease has not been reported in the cat.

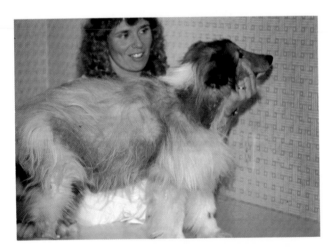

Figure 6-22 *Fourteen-year-old Shetland Sheepdog with Sertoli's cell tumor dermatopathy has alopecia and hyperpigmentation of trunk and neck.*

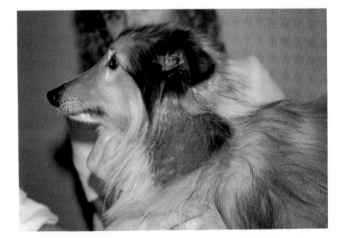

Figure 6-23 *Close-up photograph of left side of neck of Sheltie shown in Figure 6-22.*

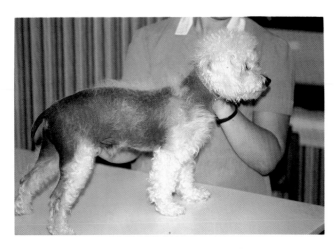

Figure 6-24   *Eleven-year-old Miniature Poodle shows extensive alopecia and hyperpigmentation.*

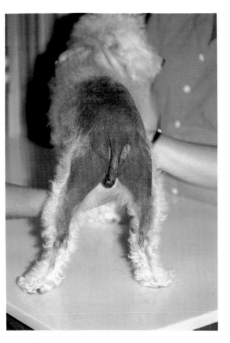

Figure 6-25   *Caudal view of Poodle shown in Figure 6-24. Patient's Sertoli's cell tumor was located in retained testicle.*

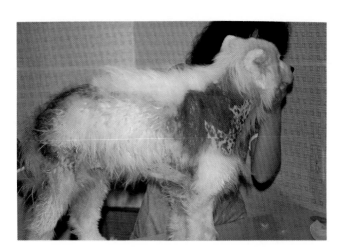

Figure 6-26   *Samoyed with marked truncal alopecia, and pigmentary abnormalities (melanosis).*

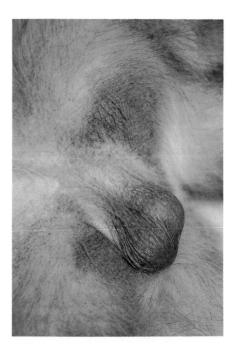

Figure 6-27   *Scrotum of patient shown in Figure 6-26. Right testicle contained palpable Sertoli's cell tumor.*

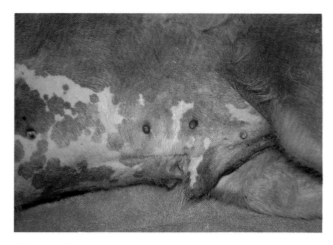

Figure 6-28 *Nine-year-old mixed-breed dog has splotchy hypopigmentation and hyperpigmentation (melanosis) of abdomen.*

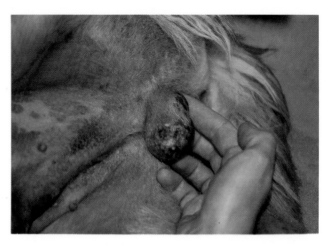

Figure 6-29 *Scrotum of patient shown in Figure 6-28 shows enlarged right testicle which contained a Sertoli's cell tumor.*

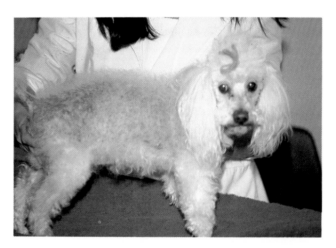

Figure 6-30 *Miniature Poodle with Sertoli's cell tumor dermatopathy shows truncal alopecia and pigmentary changes.*

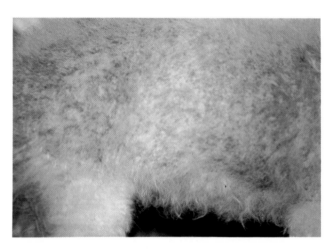

Figure 6-31 *Closer view of pigmentary changes on Poodle's skin shown in Figure 6-30.*

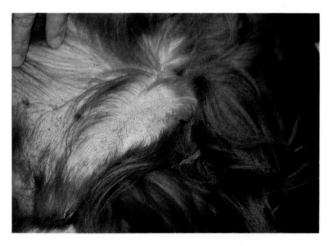

Figure 6-32 *Abdominal area of 8-year-old Irish Setter has line of erythema from scrotum extending up prepuce. This "red line" appears to be pathognomonic for Sertoli's cell tumors.*

Male Feminizing Syndrome

CLINICAL SIGNS

1. Bilaterally symmetric alopecia usually involves ventral areas and flanks
2. Seborrheic dermatitis which may be quite severe
3. Patients are often quite pruritic due to the inflammation caused by the seborrheic dermatitis
4. Ceruminous otitis may be present
5. Gynecomastia
6. Patients may sexually attract other male dogs

DIFFERENTIAL DIAGNOSIS

1. Sertoli's cell tumor dermatopathy
2. Testosterone-responsive dermatosis
3. Hypothyroidism
4. Adult-onset hyposomatotropism
5. Seborrheic dermatoses
6. Food hypersensitivity
7. Allergic inhalant disease

DIAGNOSTIC AIDS

1. Rule out other differentials
2. Skin biopsies for histopathologic examination are not diagnostic
3. It is reported that some patients respond to castration, whereas some patients respond to either testosterone or estrogen supplementation
4. Testes are normal on histopathologic examination
5. Serum levels of testosterone and estrogen are difficult to interpret

COMMENTS

Male feminizing syndrome is a rare disease affecting middle-aged intact male dogs. The underlying etiology of this disease is not known. (It may actually be a myriad of various sex hormone imbalances/hypersensitivities.) Some cases are thought to be true Sertoli's cell tumor cases that were misdiagnosed on histopathologic examination of the testes.

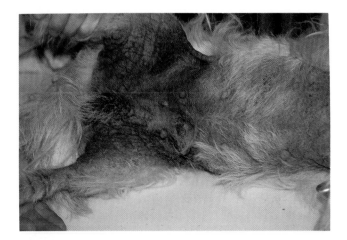

Figure 6-33 Male intact mixed-breed dog has hyperpigmentation and lichenification of inguinal area, partial alopecia of chest and gynecomastia. Patient was quite pruritic.

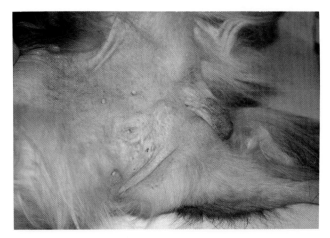

Figure 6-34 Mixed Shetland Sheepdog with alopecia, erythema, and bacterial folliculitis of abdominal and inguinal areas.

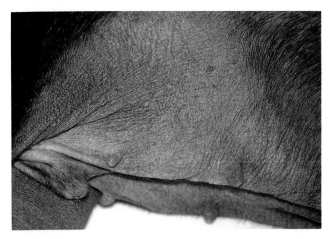

Figure 6-35 Abdominal hyperpigmentation and lichenification in adult Doberman Pinscher. Testes palpated normally, and serum sex hormone levels were normal; however, castration was curative.

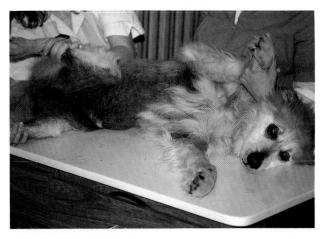

Figure 6-36 Alopecia, hyperpigmentation, and lichenification on entire ventrum of 13-year-old intact male mixed-breed dog. Castration was curative.

Testosterone-Responsive Dermatosis of Male and Female Dogs

CLINICAL SIGNS

1. Bilaterally symmetric alopecia usually involving the caudal thighs, flanks, and/or lateral thoracic areas
2. Skin in involved areas is often hyperpigmented
3. Patients are nonpruritic
4. Associated seborrheic dermatosis is uncommon

DIFFERENTIAL DIAGNOSIS

1. Hypothyroidism
2. Estrogen-responsive dermatosis

3. Sertoli's cell tumor dermatopathy
4. Adult-onset hyposomatotropism
5. Hyperadrenocorticism

DIAGNOSTIC AIDS

1. Rule out other endocrinopathies
2. Response to trial treatment with methyltestosterone
3. Serum levels of testosterone are difficult to interpret

COMMENTS

Testosterone-responsive dermatosis is an uncommon disease of middle-aged to older dogs. The condition may occur in neutered and intact males and in neutered females. The underlying etiology of this dermatosis is unknown. As with the male feminizing syndrome, this disorder may actually be a myriad of various sex hormone imbalances.

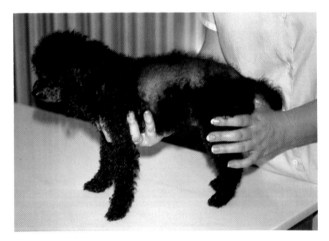

Figure 6-37 *Five-year-old female spayed Toy Poodle shows bilaterally symmetric alopecia of trunk. Skin in involved areas is hyperpigmented. Patient was nonpruritic.*

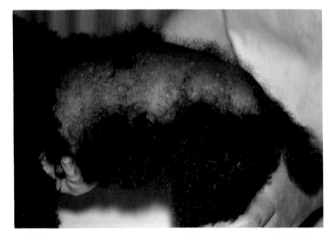

Figure 6-38 *Closer view of alopecic areas on patient shown in Figure 6-37. Treatment with low-dose, oral testosterone resulted in complete regrowth of haircoat.*

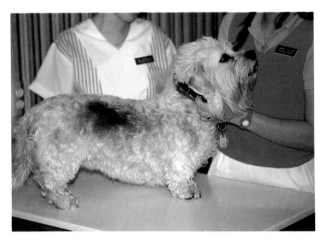

Figure 6-39 *Three-year-old female spayed Dandie Dinnmont Terrier with bilaterally symmetric alopecia of trunk.*

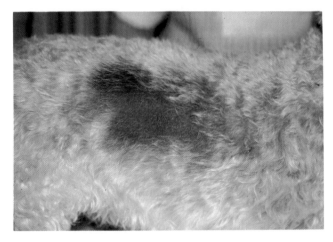

Figure 6-40 *Closer view of patient shown in Figure 6-39. Alopecic area is hyperpigmented. Patient was nonpruritic.*

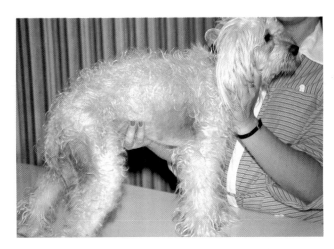

Figure 6-41   *Male altered Miniature Poodle has alopecia, with some hyperpigmentation of lateral thorax, caudal thigh, and tail. Pattern was bilaterally symmetric.*

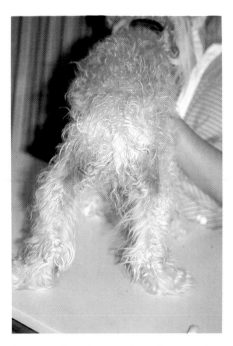

Figure 6-42   *Another view of patient shown in Figure 6-41. Patient was nonpruritic. Alopecia responded totally to oral testosterone therapy.*

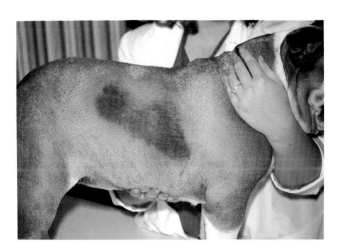

Figure 6-43   *Spayed female English Bulldog with bilaterally symmetric alopecia of lateral thorax. Alopecia responded completely to testosterone therapy but recurred when drug was discontinued.*

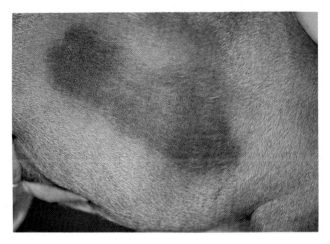

Figure 6-44   *Closer view of alopecic area on patient shown in Figure 6-43. As with all testosterone-responsive dermatoses, the patient was nonpruritic.*

Ovarian Imbalance (Hyperestrogenism in Female Dogs)

CLINICAL SIGNS

1. Bilaterally symmetric alopecia which involves the ventrum, perineal areas, caudal thighs, and/or trunk
2. Skin in involved areas may be hyperpigmented
3. Vulvar enlargement
4. Gynecomastia with or without lactation
5. Some patients develop seborrheic dermatitis and ceruminous otitis
6. Pruritus varies from moderate to nonexistent

DIFFERENTIAL DIAGNOSIS

1. Hypothyroidism
2. Hyperadrenocorticism
3. Adult-onset hyposomatotropism
4. Seborrheic dermatitis
5. Hormonal hypersensitivity

DIAGNOSTIC AIDS

1. Rule out other differentials
2. Serum levels of estrogen and progesterone may be helpful
3. Skin biopsies for histopathologic examination are nondiagnostic
4. Response to ovariohysterectomy

COMMENTS

Ovarian imbalance or hyperestrogenism is a rare disorder of the female dog. No breed predilection has been documented. Middle-aged dogs are predisposed. The disorder has not been reported in the cat.

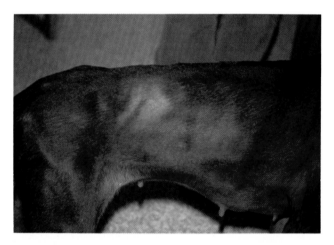

Figure 6-45 *Alopecia of flank area in young Doberman Pinscher. Alopecic pattern was bilaterally symmetric. Patient was nonpruritic.*

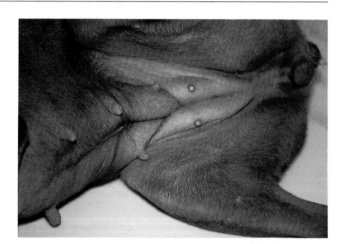

Figure 6-46 *Enlarged mammary glands of patient shown in Figure 6-45. Patient was lactating and had history of false pregnancies.*

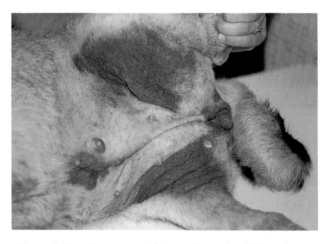

Figure 6-47 *Three-year-old intact Norwegian Elkhound shows areas of hyperpigmentation and lichenification.*

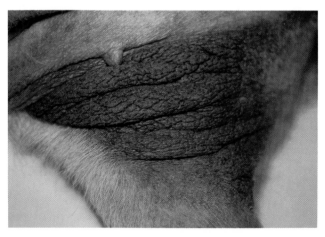

Figure 6-48 *Closer view of medial thigh of patient shown in Figure 6-47. Ovariohysterectomy was curative.*

Estrogen-Responsive Dermatosis of Male and Female Dogs

CLINICAL SIGNS

1. Bilaterally symmetric alopecia usually involving the ventrum, perineal areas, caudal thighs, trunk, and/or ear pinnae
2. Skin in involved areas may be slightly hyperpigmented
3. Patients are nonpruritic

DIFFERENTIAL DIAGNOSIS

1. Testosterone-responsive dermatosis
2. Hypothyroidism
3. Hyperadrenocorticism
4. Adult-onset hyposomatotropism

DIAGNOSTIC AIDS

1. Rule out other endocrinopathies
2. Response to trial therapy with low-dose oral diethylstilbestrol

COMMENTS

Estrogen-responsive dermatosis is an uncommon disorder of neutered male and female dogs. No age, breed, or sex predilection has been documented. The disorder has not been reported in the cat. Care must be exercised in treating dogs with exogenous estrogens since severe, life-threatening side effects are possible.

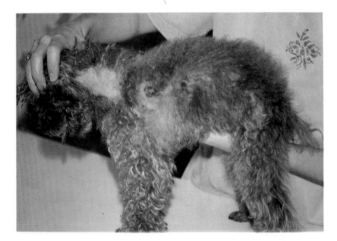

Figure 6-49   *Seven-year-old female spayed Toy Poodle has marked alopecia of neck and lateral thoracic areas. Patient was nonpruritic.*

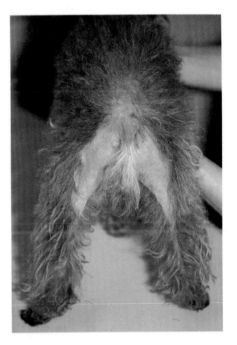

Figure 6-50   *Another view of patient shown in Figure 6-49. Alopecia was completely responsive to very low dose of oral diethylstilbestrol.*

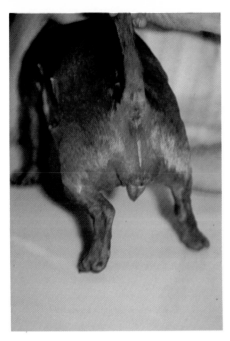

Figure 6-51 *Perineal area of 4-year-old female spayed Short-Haired Miniature Dachshund. Alopecic pattern developed 2 years after ovariohysterectomy.*

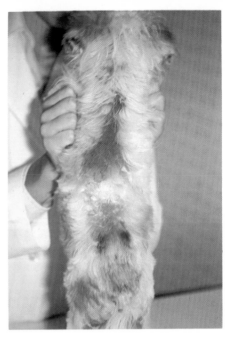

Figure 6-52 *Areas of alopecia and hyperpigmentation on dorsal midline of female spayed mixed-breed dog.*

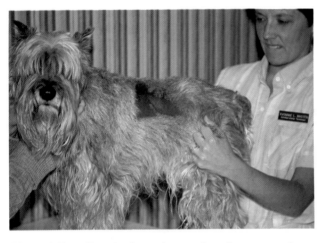

Figure 6-53 *Alopecic, hyperpigmented patch on neutered male Miniature Schnauzer. Treatment with low-dose oral diethylstilbestrol resulted in normal regrowth of hair.*

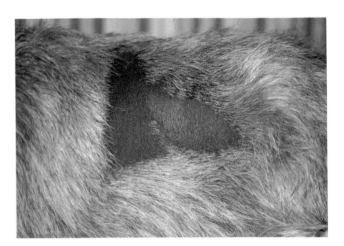

Figure 6-54 *Close-up photograph of alopecic area on patient shown in Figure 6-53.*

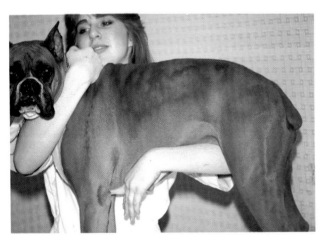

Figure 6-55 *Patchy alopecia with hyperpigmentation on lateral thorax of 8-year-old neutered male Boxer.*

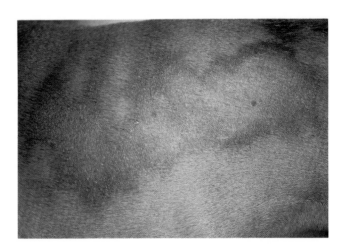

Figure 6-56 *Closer view of alopecic patch on patient shown in Figure 6-53.*

Canine Hypothyroidism

CLINICAL SIGNS

1. Bilaterally symmetric alopecia which may involve all areas of the body except the distal extremities
2. Alopecia on the bridge of the nose is a common finding in severe cases
3. Dull, dry, and brittle coat
4. Easy epilation of hair
5. Hyperpigmentation of skin in involved areas is common
6. Skin often feels thick and puffy
7. Seborrheic dermatosis and ceruminous otitis are found in approximately 25% of hypothyroid patients
8. Lowered resistance to bacterial skin infections
9. Delayed wound healing
10. Acral pruritic nodules (lick granulomas)
11. Pruritus exists only when secondary bacterial dermatitis and/or seborrheic dermatoses are present
12. Patients may also suffer from lethargy, personality changes, obesity, and thermophilia
13. Some patients have a tragic or worried facial expression
14. In addition to the above clinical signs, various ocular, reproductive, cardiovascular, gastrointestinal, and neuromuscular abnormalities may be present

DIFFERENTIAL DIAGNOSIS

1. Hyperadrenocorticism
2. Adult-onset hyposomatotropism
3. Testosterone-responsive dermatopathy
4. Estrogen-responsive dermatopathy
5. Other causes of seborrheic and bacterial dermatitis

DIAGNOSTIC AIDS

1. Resting serum levels of total T_4, free T_4, total T_3, and free T_3
2. Thyroid-stimulating hormone (TSH) response testing
3. Serum levels of thyroid-stimulating hormone
4. Complete blood count may reveal a normochromic, normocytic, nonregenerative anemia
5. Serum cholesterol is often elevated

COMMENTS

Hypothyroidism is the most common canine endocrine imbalance. Many breeds are reported to be "predisposed" to develop hypothyroidism. The author has found the highest incidence of the disease in the Great Dane, Golden Retriever, Doberman Pinscher, and Chow Chow. No sex predilection has been documented. The average age at diagnosis of the disease is between 6 and 11 years.

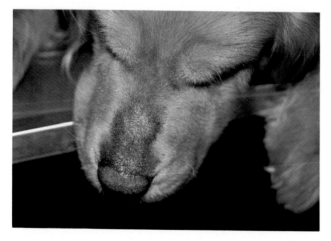

Figure 6-57 *Three-year-old Golden Retriever shows obvious lethargy, worried look, and alopecia of bridge of nose.*

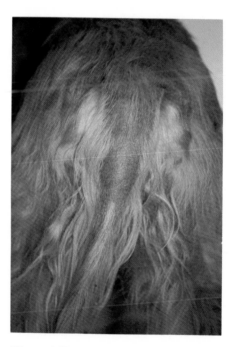

Figure 6-58 *Caudal view of patient shown in Figure 6-57. Note alopecia with hyperpigmentation of tail, rump, and caudal thighs.*

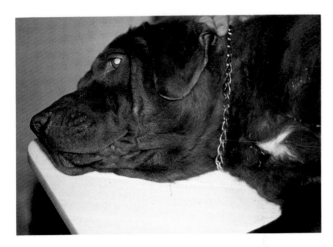

Figure 6-59 *Four-year-old overweight Chocolate Labrador Retriever shows thick, puffy jowls. Patient was quite lethargic.*

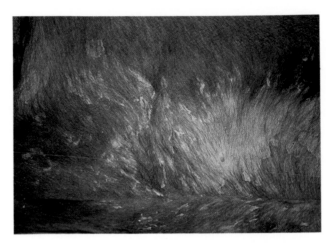

Figure 6-60 *Ventral chest of patient shown in Figure 6-59. Note thinning haircoat, healing bacterial dermatitis, and scaling.*

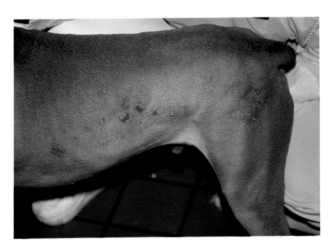

Figure 6-61 *Patchy alopecia and bacterial dermatitis on lateral thorax and flank of adult hypothyroid Boxer.*

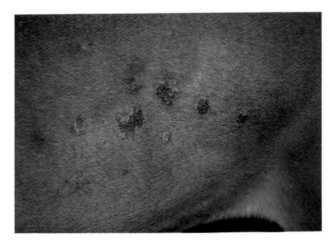

Figure 6-62 *Closer view of bacterial lesions shown in Figure 6-61.*

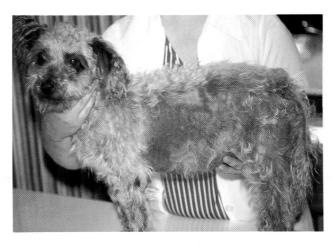

Figure 6-63 *Marked alopecia with some hyperpigmentation on trunk of 10-year-old mixed-breed hypothyroid dog.*

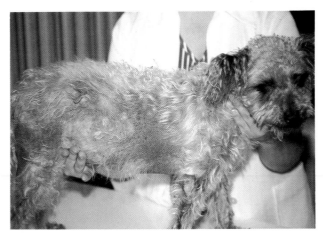

Figure 6-64 *Right side of patient shown in Figure 6-63.*

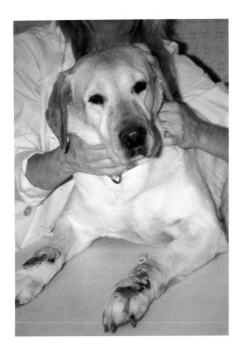

Figure 6-65 *Four-year-old, overweight, lethargic, male yellow Labrador Retriever. Note numerous acral pruritic nodules (lick granulomas) on patient's forelegs.*

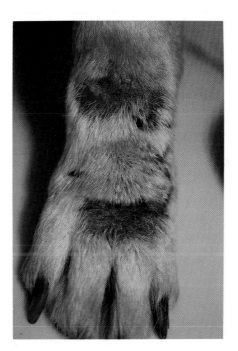

Figure 6-66 *Closer view of acral pruritic nodules on foreleg of patient shown in Figure 6-65. Lesions responded completely to thyroid replacement therapy.*

Feline Hypothyroidism

CLINICAL SIGNS

1. Alopecia may involve the trunk and/or neck
2. Some patients have seborrhea sicca which may be the only obvious clinical sign
3. Truncal hair may epilate easily
4. Patients are nonpruritic

DIFFERENTIAL DIAGNOSIS

1. Self-induced alopecia including allergic and neurodermatoses
2. Other causes of seborrhea sicca

DIAGNOSTIC AIDS

1. Blood samples for resting total T_4, free T_4, total T_3 and free T_3
2. Skin biopsies for histopathologic examination are helpful but not diagnostic

COMMENTS

Hypothyroidism is rare in the cat. It is frequently overdiagnosed because many feline skin diseases result in self-induced alopecia which may resemble an "endocrine" pattern.

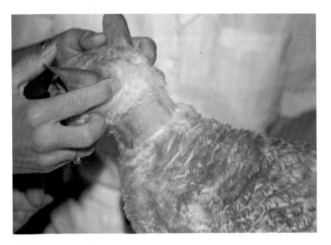

Figure 6-67 *Five-year-old female spayed Cornish Rex cat shows alopecia around neck which involves the entire circumference.*

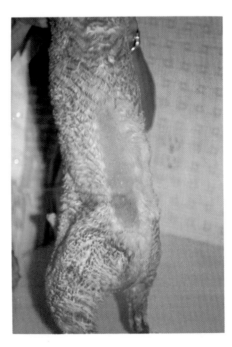

Figure 6-68 *Another view of patient shown in Figure 6-67 shows truncal alopecia. Cat had very low free T_4 levels and showed complete regrowth of hair after thyroid supplementation.*

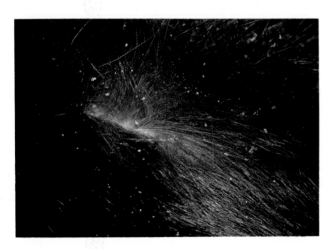

Figure 6-69 *Seborrhea sicca on trunk of 7-year-old female spayed hypothroid cat.*

Feline Hyperthyroidism

CLINICAL SIGNS

1. Excessive grooming, which results in self-induced alopecia of any part of the body, especially the abdomen, lateral thoracic areas, and legs
2. Hyperactivity and restlessness are common signs
3. Continual walking and frequent crying are common
4. Patients are often thin despite a voracious appetite
5. Tachycardia and various arrhythmias may be detected
6. A mass may be found on thyroid palpation

DIFFERENTIAL DIAGNOSIS

1. Flea bite hypersensitivity*
2. Food hypersensitivity*
3. Allergic inhalant disease*
4. Psychogenic alopecia*

All causes of self-induced alopecia must be considered.

DIAGNOSTIC AIDS

1. Serum levels of L-thyroxine (T_4) and/or triiodothyronine(T_3) are elevated
2. Palpating mass in thyroid area of the neck

COMMENTS

Hyperthyroidism is a rare cause of self-induced alopecia in the cat. Older cats, greater than 9 years of age, are predisposed. No breed or sex predilection has been documented. The cause of hyperthyroidism in 90% of feline patients is either adenomatous hyperplasia or adenomas. The other 10% suffer from adenocarcinomas.

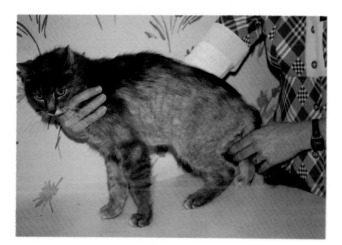

Figure 6-70 Severe self-induced alopecia on trunk and rear legs of 8-year-old Domestic Short-Haired cat. Hair loss pattern was bilaterally symmetric. Haircoat completely regrew after removal of thyroid adenoma.

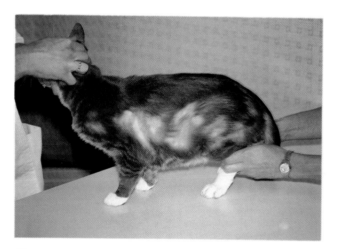

Figure 6-71 Self-induced alopecia on shoulder, lateral thorax, and rump of 10-year-old hyperthyroid cat.

Canine Hypoadrenocorticism (Addison's Disease)

CLINICAL SIGNS

1. The only cutaneous abnormalities that this author has recognized in Addisonian patients is an abnormally long haircoat that is lighter in color than the patient's original, preaddisonian coat
2. Noncutaneous signs include depression, weakness, anorexia, shivering, diarrhea, vomiting, weight loss, abdominal pain, polydipsia, polyuria, and reluctance to walk

DIFFERENTIAL DIAGNOSIS

1. Hypertrichosis has been reported in some hypothyroid dogs
2. Numerous gastrointestinal and renal diseases have similar noncutaneous signs

DIAGNOSTIC AIDS

1. Serum electrolytes are abnormal; hyponatremia, hypochloremia, and hyperkalemia
2. Electrocardiogram changes consistent with hyperkalemia are common findings
3. Measurement of plasma cortisol
4. Adrenocorticotropic hormone (ACTH) stimulation tests
5. Plasma adrenocorticotropic hormone levels

COMMENTS

An abnormally long haircoat associated with Addison's disease has not been reported in the dog. The author has seen three cases in which the patients had abnormally long haircoats that were lighter in color than the original coats. The abnormal coats appeared to be directly related to the development of Addison's disease in these patients. No other cutaneous abnormalities were present. Once the disease was corrected and the abnormally long hair was shed, the coats grew in a normal length. Hypoadrenocorticism appears to be a disease of young and middle-aged dogs. No breed or sex predilections have been documented. Addison's disease has not been reported in the cat.

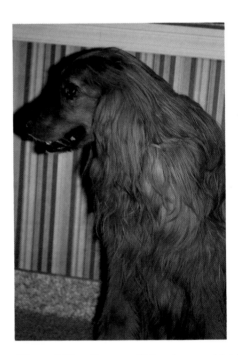

Figure 6-72 Six-year-old female spayed Irish Setter with Addison's disease. Only cutaneous abnormality was exceptionally long haircoat, which was lighter in color than patient's original haircoat. Some hairs on patient's head were over 12 inches long.

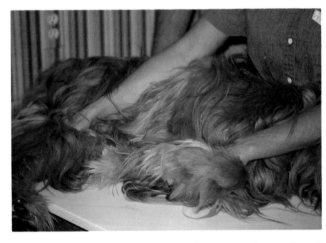

Figure 6-73 Note abnormally long haircoat on legs and trunk of patient shown in Figure 6-72.

FUNGAL INFECTIONS

Canine Dermatophyte Infection (Superficial Fungal Infection, Dermatophytosis, Ringworm)

CLINICAL SIGNS

1. Circular patches of alopecia on any part of the body
2. Varying degrees of seborrheic dermatoses
3. Crusts and/or hyperkeratotic plaques
4. Erythematous plaques
5. Folliculitis that resembles bacterial folliculitis
6. Some patients develop kerions, which are inflamed nodules often with secondary bacterial infection
7. Pruritus is variable but most frequently is mild to nonexistent

DIFFERENTIAL DIAGNOSIS

1. Demodicosis
2. Bacterial dermatitis
3. Seborrheic dermatitis
4. Contact dermatitis
5. Pemphigus foliaceus

DIAGNOSTIC AIDS

1. Diagnosis should *never* be based upon clinical signs since dermatophytosis resembles many canine skin diseases
2. Most *Microsporum canis* infections will fluoresce an apple green color under Wood's light examination. This diagnostic test may be misleading since many seborrheic and other skin abnormalities "fluoresce" a bluish color
3. Fungal culture is the most accurate way to diagnose dermatophyte infections. It is important to stain and microscopically identify any growth that occurs within 14 days on fungal cultures. Growth on fungal culture media does *not* necessarily mean that the patient has a dermatophyte infection

COMMENTS

Canine "ringworm" is the most overdiagnosed canine skin disease. It is absolutely essential to culture and to determine that the growth on a fungal culture media is a true dermatophyte before making a diagnosis of dermatophyte infection. The most common causative agents in canine dermatophyte infection are *Microsporum canis*, *Microsporum gypseum*, and *Trichophyton mentagrophytes*.

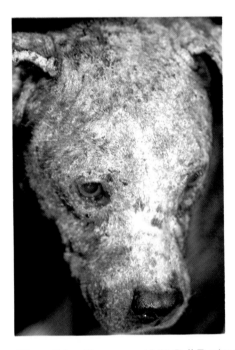

Figure 7-1 *Three-year-old Pit Bull Terrier with near-total alopecia of face, head, and ears. Note extensive scaling, crusting, and excoriated papules.*

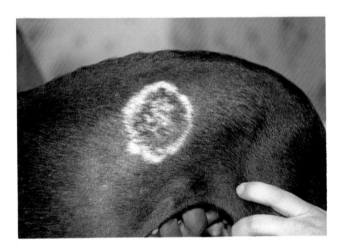

Figure 7-2 *Lesion on flank of patient shown in Figure 7-1. This circular rim of alopecia with central "healing" is classic dermatophyte lesion; however, other clinical manifestations of dermatophytosis are much more common.*

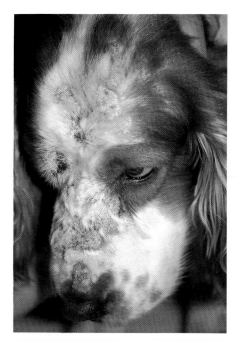

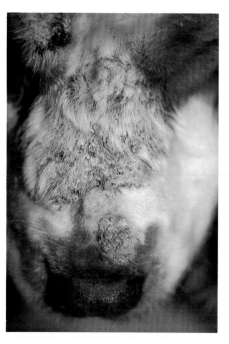

Figure 7-3 *Alopecic, crusted lesions on face and head of 2-year-old Welsh Springer Spaniel with severe, generalized* Microsporum canis *infection.*

Figure 7-4 *Closer view of lesions shown in Figure 7-3.*

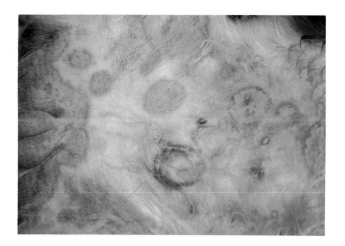

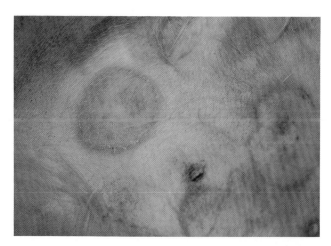

Figure 7-5 *Abdominal and inguinal areas of patient shown in Figures 7-3 and 7-4. These circular, erythematous lesions resemble bacterial hypersensitivity and bacterial hypersensitivity–like lesions.*

Figure 7-6 *Closer view of lesions shown in Figure 7-5.*

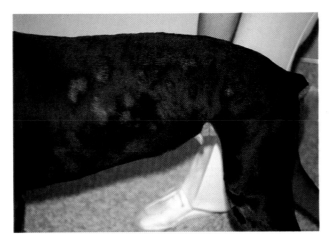

Figure 7-7 *Patchy, circular areas of alopecia on trunk of 15-month-old Doberman Pinscher. Lesions were not pruritic.*

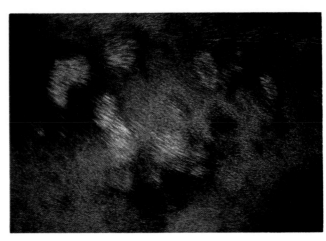

Figure 7-8 *Closer view of lesions shown in Figure 7-7. These lesions may be mistaken for bacterial folliculitis.*

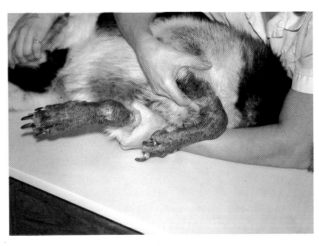

Figure 7-9 *Alopecic, hyperpigmented, scaling forelegs of 11-year-old German Shepherd dog with* Trichophyton mentagrophytes *dermatophytosis.*

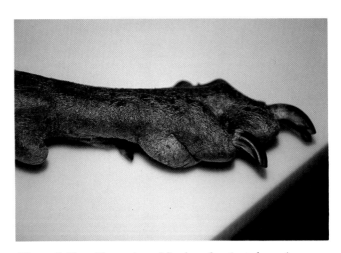

Figure 7-10 *Closer view of foreleg of patient shown in Figure 7-9.*

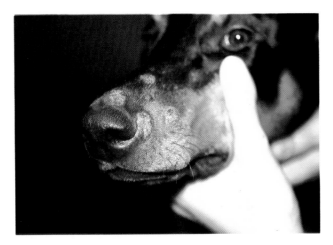

Figure 7-11 *Fungal kerions on muzzle of young Doberman Pinscher. This* Microsporum canis *infection was acquired via direct contact with infected kitten.*

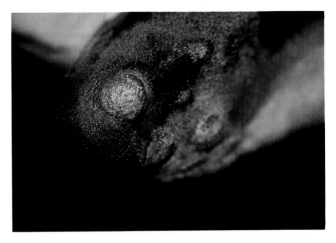

Figure 7-12 *Closer view of kerion shown in Figure 7-11.*

Feline Dermatophyte Infection (Superficial Fungal Infection, Dermatophytosis, Ringworm)

CLINICAL SIGNS

1. Circular areas of alopecia often with mild erythema on any part of the body but most frequently on the head and face
2. Miliary dermatitis consisting of papules with or without excoriations usually located on the mid-back
3. Self-induced alopecia
4. Head and neck excoriations
5. Rarely lesions of the eosinophilic granuloma complex are caused by dermatophytes
6. Pruritus is quite variable
7. Cats, especially long-haired ones, are frequently asymptomatic carriers

DIFFERENTIAL DIAGNOSIS

1. Flea bite hypersensitivity
2. Allergic inhalant disease
3. Food hypersensitivity
4. Notoedric mange
5. Cheyletiella dermatitis
6. Demodicosis
7. Bacterial folliculitis
8. Psychogenic alopecia

DIAGNOSTIC AIDS

1. Diagnosis should *never* be based upon clinical signs since dermatophyte infection may resemble virtually any feline skin disease
2. About 50% of feline dermatophytes (for example, most of the *Microsporum canis* infections) will fluoresce under Wood's light. It is important to note that true fluoresence is an apple green color. Any scaling of the skin or skin debris will fluoresce a bluish color which may be misleading.
3. Skin biopsies for histopathologic examination may be diagnostic
4. The most accurate way to diagnose a dermatophyte infection is via fungal culture. Any growth on the culture media should be stained and examined microscopically to determine whether or not it is a true dermatophyte

COMMENTS

Dermatophyte skin infection is a common cause of feline skin disease. However, it is very frequently overdiagnosed because of misinterpreted Wood's light examinations and "positive" fungal cultures. It is the author's belief that any feline skin disease (pruritic or nonpruritic) should be cultured for fungal infection and that no cat should be treated for dermatophytosis unless a fungal culture is positive and the causative organism is identified. The most common feline dermatophytes are *Microsporum canis*, *Microsporum gypseum*, and *Trichophyton mentagrophytes*.

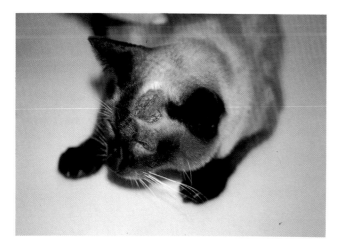

Figure 7-13 *Circular, ulcerated lesion on head of elderly Siamese cat. Culture of this lesion grew* Microsporum canis. *This patient apparently became infected with the dermatophyte during cat fight.*

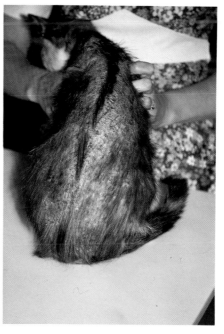

Figure 7-14 *Extensive alopecia with broken hairs and miliary dermatitis on trunk of 5-year-old Calico cat. This patient's* Microsporum canis *dermatophytosis was quite pruritic.*

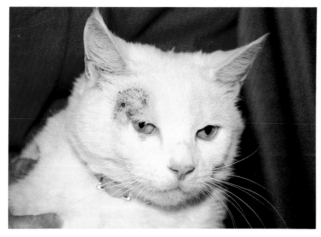

Figure 7-15 Microsporum gypseum *dermatophytosis manifested by circular area of partial alopecia and crusting in preauricular area of middle-aged Domestic Short-Haired cat.*

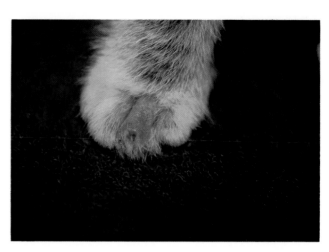

Figure 7-16 *Alopecic, erythematous lesions on forefoot of 9-week-old kitten caused by* Microsporum canis *infection.*

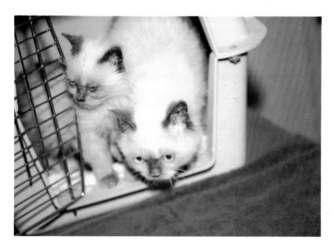

Figure 7-17 *Eight-week-old Himalayan kittens with asymptomatic* Microsporum canis *infection. These kittens were presented for examination because two family members had developed dermatophyte infections.*

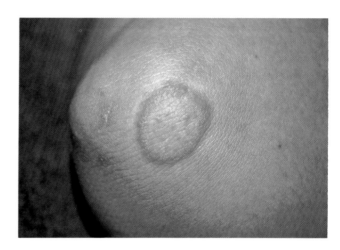

Figure 7-18 *Dermatophyte lesion on elbow of female teenage owner of kittens shown in Figure 7-17.*

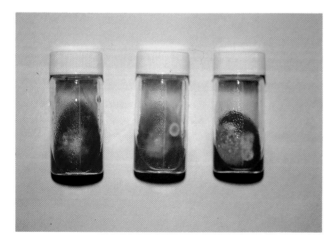

Figure 7-19 *Fungal cultures taken from feline skin lesions. Bottle on left grew* Microsporum canis. *Other two bottles grew nonpathogenic fungi. It is important to note that change in phenol red color indicator from yellow to red does* not *necessarily mean that the fungus is a dermatophyte.*

Candidiasis

CLINICAL SIGNS

1. Grayish white plaques may appear on mucous membranes (or less commonly skin) surrounded by marked erythema
2. The most common site of infection is the oral mucosa
3. Other sites of infection include the nail beds, vagina, prepuce, anus, and external ear canal
4. Skin involvement is rare
5. Oral lesions are frequently accompanied by a very obvious foul odor that is usually the presenting complaint

DIFFERENTIAL DIAGNOSIS

1. Ulcerative diseases of the oral cavity including pemphigus vulgaris
2. Acute moist dermatitis
3. Vulvar fold dermatitis
4. Bacterial or fungal otitis externa
5. Dermatophilosis

DIAGNOSTIC AIDS

1. Cultures of exudate on Sabouraud's dextrose agar without cycloheximide
2. Budding cells and pseudohyphae may be seen on stained smears of exudate but careful identification is very important
3. Mucosa and/or skin biopsies for histopathologic examination are often helpful but may not be diagnostic

COMMENTS

Candidiasis is an infection caused by *Candida* species. It is an uncommon cause of oral mucosa inflammation, ulceration, and odor. The infection is even less frequently seen in other mucocutaneous locations and nail beds. Skin involvement is rare. Candidiasis may be more common in immunocompromised patients and in patients receiving high dose corticosteroids and long-term antibiotics. No breed or sex predilection has been documented. Very old patients may be predisposed.

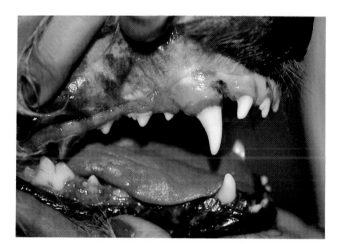

Figure 7-20 *Whitish plaques and papules on tongue and gums of Irish Wolfhound presented for halitosis. Culture of these lesions grew* Candida albicans.

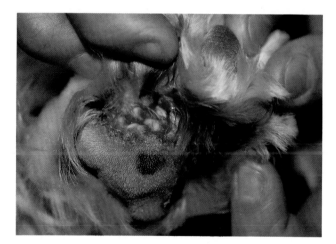

Figure 7-21 *Interdigital candidiasis in patient receiving immunosuppressive therapy for systemic lupus erythematosus.*

Malassezia Infection (*Malassezia pachydermatitis* Infection, *Pityrosporum canis* Infection)

CLINICAL SIGNS

1. Ceruminous otitis with a brown to grey exudate. The excessive cerumen production caused by the yeast frequently results in inflammation and pruritus
2. *Malassezia* has infrequently been associated with interdigital inflammation and pruritus as well as truncal dermatitis

DIFFERENTIAL DIAGNOSIS

1. Other causes of otitis externa including Cocker and Springer Spaniel seborrheic dermatitis/otitis, food hypersensitivity, flea bite hypersensitivity, and allergic inhalant disease
2. Other causes of interdigital inflammation including demodicosis, contact dermatitis, allergic inhalant disease, and food hypersensitivity

DIAGNOSTIC AIDS

1. Finding large numbers of *Malassezia pachydermatitis* on cytology of ear swab samples
2. Swabs of interdigital spaces may also show large numbers of *Malassezia*

COMMENTS

Malassezia pachydermatitis is a yeast that is a normal inhabitant of approximately 30% of canine external ear canals. This yeast has also been reported to be normal "flora" in skin folds, especially interdigital spaces. Therefore finding *Malassezia* on cytologies from these areas is often helpful but not necessarily diagnostic. Most cases of *Malassezia* otitis and dermatitis are considered to be secondary to numerous underlying etiologies. These include otic and cutaneous inflammation caused by allergic diseases and alteration of normal flora caused by antibiotics (local and systemic) and other drugs.

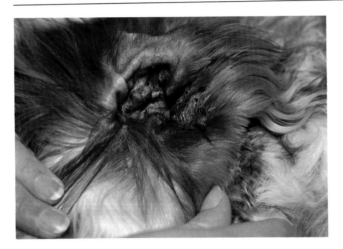

Figure 7-22   *Otitis externa in English Setter caused by* Malassezia pachydermatitis. *Note inflammation of external ear canal and brownish black, waxy discharge.*

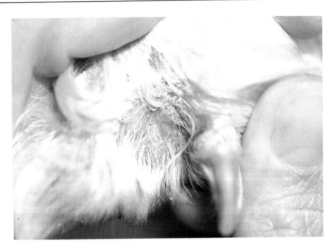

Figure 7-23   *Interdigital inflammation and seborrheic debris caused by Malassezia infection.*

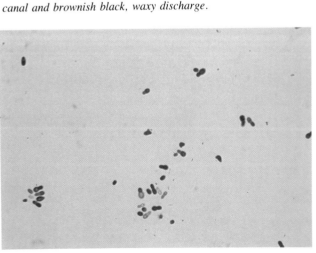

Figure 7-24   *Photomicrograph of* Malassezia pachydermatitis *in smear of exudate taken from case of otitis externa and stained with Diff Quick.*

Aspergillosis

CLINICAL SIGNS

1. The most common clinical sign is a nasal discharge (often unilateral) with a history of sneezing
2. Cutaneous signs are various forms of granulomas and ulcers and are usually manifestations of systemic disease
3. Other signs include diarrhea, weight loss, and ocular and neurologic abnormalities

DIFFERENTIAL DIAGNOSIS

1. Sporotrichosis
2. Protothecosis
3. Other mycotic infections
4. Bacterial dermatitis and sinusitis
5. Neoplasia

DIAGNOSTIC AIDS

1. Diagnosis is best made by both histopathology and positive cultures

2. Histopathologic examination of biopsy specimens should reveal tissue invasion by septate hyphae accompanied by diffuse or nodular dermatitis or by necrosis with minimal inflammation
3. Biopsy material or exudate should be cultured at room temperature on Sabouraud's dextrose agar with or without antibiotics
4. Bacterial cultures should also be performed
5. Wet mounts may demonstrate septate hyphae and *Aspergillus* conidiophores

COMMENTS

Aspergillosis is a wide group of diseases caused by *Aspergillus* species, mainly *Aspergillus fumigatus* and *Aspergillus flavus*. Since *Aspergillus* species are the most common fungi in the environment, they are very frequent laboratory contaminants. Therefore, when *Aspergillus* is found on culture it is necessary to determine if it is a pathogen or contaminant. Since these fungi are usually opportunistic, secondary invaders, they are often found in conjunction with bacterial, neoplastic, or immunosuppressive diseases.

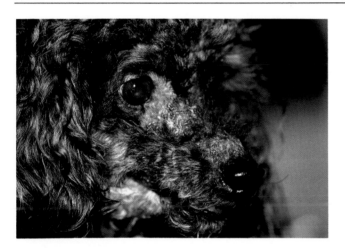

Figure 7-25   *Ulcerated nodules on face of 15-year-old Poodle with disseminated aspergillosis.*

Mycetoma (Fungal Tumor)

CLINICAL SIGNS

1. The most common sites of involvement are the feet and distal extremities; however, any area of the body may be involved
2. The earliest sign is usually subcutaneous swelling produced by fungi or bacteria in the tissue
3. These swellings are usually painful and not pruritic
4. Draining fistulous tracts soon develop
5. The exudate characteristically contains granules that are usually black in color, although they may be yellow or white

DIFFERENTIAL DIAGNOSIS

1. Phaeohyphomycosis
2. Foreign body fistula
3. Abscess
4. Neoplasm

DIAGNOSTIC AIDS

1. Wet mount potassium hydroxide preparation of exudate to show hyphae or chlamydospores
2. Wet mount Gram stain of exudate will reveal gram-positive filaments
3. Biopsies for histopathologic examination reveal diffuse or nodular dermatitis with fungal elements (grains) These fungal elements are frequently in the center of necrotic granulomatous reaction
4. Culture exudate on plain Sabouraud's dextrose agar is often diagnostic
5. It is important to differentiate between actinomycotic and eumycotic infections since treatment varies based on type of infection

COMMENTS

Mycetomas are tumefactions with draining tracts and granules present in the exudate. The infection develops when a fungus or bacteria gains entry through the skin by an injury. Causative fungi are common soil saprophytes and plant pathogens and are classified into two groups, actinomycotic and eumycotic. Actinomycotic agents include various species of *Actinomyces*, *Nocardia*, *Actinomadura*, and *Streptomyces*. Eumycotic agents include *Curvularia geniculata*, *Allescheria boydii*, and *Madurella* species. A variety of soil bacteria have also been demonstrated to cause mycetomas.

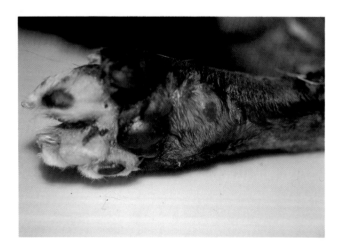

Figure 7-26   *Area of inflammation with some ulceration proximal to metatarsal pad in a 6-year-old Domestic Short-Haired cat. Lesion was mildly pruritic and quite painful.*

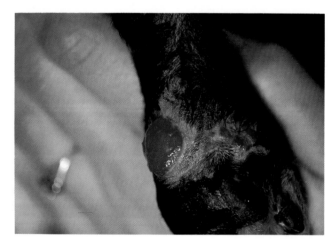

Figure 7-27   *Ulcerated nodule with draining tracts on forefoot of 2-year-old Domestic Short-Haired cat.*

Phaeohyphomycosis

CLINICAL SIGNS

1. Early lesions are painless nodules in the subcutis
2. Fistulas typically form in the nodules and a purulent, pink or yellow exudate may be present
3. Ulceration of the lesions is common
4. Lesions may be cutaneous, subcutaneous, and/or systemic

DIFFERENTIAL DIAGNOSIS

1. Foreign body fistulas
2. Chronic abscesses
3. Deep pyoderma
4. Mycetomas
5. Ulcerative diseases such as bullous pemphigoid and toxic epidermal necrolysis
6. Neoplasia
7. Feline leprosy

DIAGNOSTIC AIDS

1. Fungal culture of the exudate or of tissue pieces is diagnostic. The media is plain Sabouraud's without antibiotics or cycloheximide
2. Skin biopsies for histopathologic examination to reveal diffuse or nodular dermatitis and fungal elements

COMMENTS

Phaeohyphomycosis is a rare fungal disease of the dog and cat. The organisms are commonly found in soil, on plants, and in the air. Most are considered to be saprophytes and are generally of low pathogenicity to animals and man. Some patients have been shown to have compromised immune systems. One must be extremely careful in making a diagnosis of phaeohyphomycosis because the causative organisms are commonly found in "nature" and are frequently laboratory contaminants.

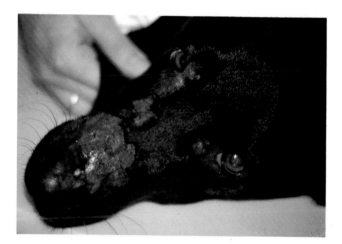

Figure 7-28 Coalescing ulcerated nodules on face of young mixed Labrador Retriever. Culture of biopsy specimens revealed phaeohyphomycosis.

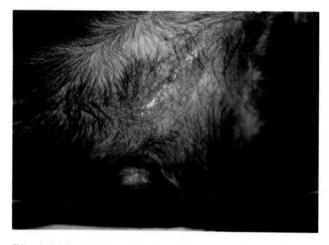

Figure 7-29 Ulcerated, draining lesions on abdomen of patient shown in Figure 7-28. Lesions were nonpruritic and nonpainful.

Protothecosis

CLINICAL SIGNS

1. Cutaneous lesions reported in dogs include granulomas and dry, crusted patches. Nasal exudate has also been reported
2. In cats the only reported cutaneous lesions are soft, fluctuant, subcutaneous masses
3. Signs of other organ involvement include polydipsia, polyuria, polyphagia, chronic nephritis, hemorrhagic diarrhea, and iritis

DIFFERENTIAL DIAGNOSIS

1. Sporotrichosis
2. Foreign body granulomas
3. Mycetoma
4. Phaeohyphomycosis
5. Neoplasia

DIAGNOSTIC AIDS

1. Culture exudate on Sabouraud's dextrose agar or blood agar with or without antibiotics
2. Microscopic examination of potassium hydroxide preparations of exudate to reveal oval to globose structures containing two or more autospores

COMMENTS

Protothecosis is a systemic and/or cutaneous disease caused by various species of *Prototheca*, mainly *Prototheca wickerhamii*. *Prototheca* species have been found in water, soil, human feces, and sewage. Possible routes of transmission to animals include cutaneous injury, inhalation, and ingestion.

Photos to illustrate this disease were not available prior to publication.

Sporotrichosis

CLINICAL SIGNS

1. The most common clinical signs are nodules, granulomas, and shallow ulcers
2. The nodules are usually alopecic, circumscribed, and nonpainful
3. These lesions may follow the lymphatic pathways on the extremities or they may be spread randomly over the body
4. A reddish brown discharge may be present if the nodules rupture
5. The disease may be disseminated with multiple organ involvement, especially of the lungs and liver

DIFFERENTIAL DIAGNOSIS

1. Deep pyodermas
2. Chronic ulcers
3. Feline leprosy
4. Other mycoses such as histoplasmosis, cryptococcosis, blastomycosis, phaeohyphomycosis, and mycetomas

DIAGNOSTIC AIDS

1. Culture exudate or biopsy specimens on Sabouraud's dextrose agar or brain-heart infusion agar
2. *Sporothrix schenckii* organisms are very difficult to find on histopathologic examination of biopsy specimens except in feline samples
3. Direct examination of exudate in potassium hydroxide preparations rarely reveals the organisms

COMMENTS

Sporothrix schenckii is a soil saprophyte that may invade the skin of dogs and cats by puncture wounds or wound contamination. In some cases the organism has caused disease by inhalation or ingestion. Sporotrichosis may be transmitted from animals to man if the exudate from infected animals comes in contact with open wounds or scratches on human skin.

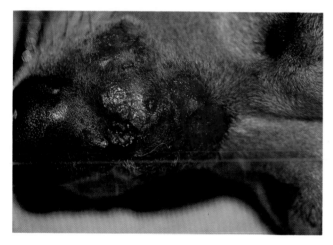

Figure 7-30   *Ulcerated coalescing nodules on muzzle of 7-year-old mixed-breed dog. Culture of biopsy specimens revealed* Sporothrix schenckii.

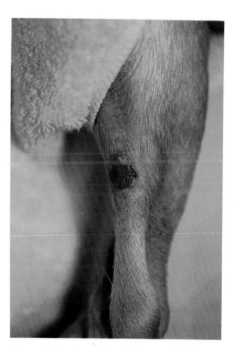

Figure 7-31   *Ulcerated lesion on right rear leg of patient shown in Figure 7-30. Ulcerated lesions were present on two other limbs.*

Blastomycosis

CLINICAL SIGNS

1. The most common cutaneous signs are cutaneous and subcutaneous abscesses, draining tracts, ulcers, and granulomas
2. Popliteal and prescapular lymph nodes may be enlarged and draining
3. Other signs include anorexia, depression, respiratory disease, often including a cough and dyspnea, exophthalmia, lameness, prostatitis, and testicular abnormalities

DIFFERENTIAL DIAGNOSIS

1. Other systemic mycoses such as coccidioidomycosis, histoplasmosis, and cryptococcosis
2. Disseminated neoplastic disease may resemble blastomycosis

DIAGNOSTIC AIDS

1. Wet mounts of exudate from skin lesions in potassium hydroxide and India ink or new methylene blue reveal large, thick-walled, budding yeasts with double contoured walls
2. Agar gel immunodiffusion test
3. Histopathologic examination of biopsy specimens reveal budding yeasts surrounded by a pyogranulomatous reaction

COMMENTS

Blastomycosis is a multisystemic disease caused by the dimorphic fungus *Blastomyces dermatitidis*. The disease affects primarily dogs and man. Young, male dogs appear to be at higher risk. The disease has been reported less frequently in the cat. Siamese cats may be predisposed. *Blastomyces dermatitidis* has been isolated from soil rich in organic matter; however, the source of most infections is unknown. Infection usually occurs following the inhalation of spores.

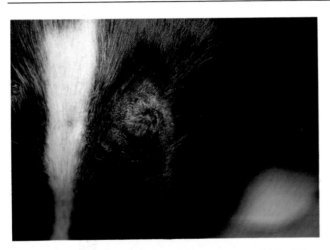

Figure 7-32 *Draining nodule on head of 2-year-old English Springer Spaniel. Wet mount of exudate revealed thick-walled, budding yeasts with double contoured walls.*

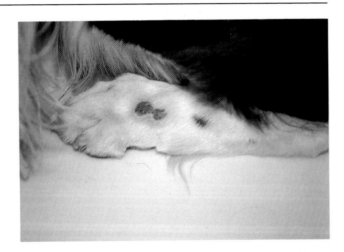

Figure 7-33 *Left forefoot of patient shown in Figure 7-32.*

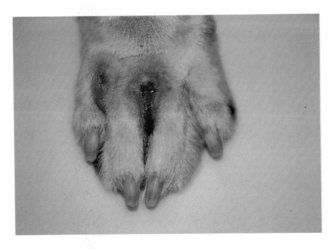

Figure 7-34 *Forefoot of patient shown in Figures 7-32 and 7-33. Stained exudate from this lesion also revealed* Blastomyces dermatitidis.

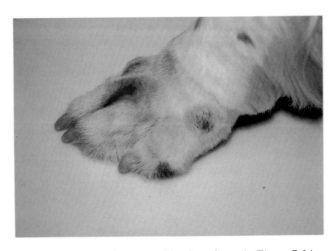

Figure 7-35 *Another view of forefoot shown in Figure 7-34. Entire foot was swollen and quite painful.*

Coccidioidomycosis (Valley Fever)

CLINICAL SIGNS

1. Coccidioidomycosis is divided into either a primary or disseminated form. The primary form may be either cutaneous or pulmonary. Primary cutaneous disease is rare
2. Cutaneous disease is manifested by firm, painless nodules with central ulceration and by regional lymphadenitis and lymphadenopathy
3. Pulmonary disease may be manifested by tracheobronchitis or may be asymptomatic
4. Signs of disseminated disease include fever, cough, dyspnea, anorexia, weight loss, depression, lameness, and peripheral lymphadenopathy with or without abscessation

DIFFERENTIAL DIAGNOSIS

1. Other systemic mycoses such as blastomycosis, histoplasmosis, and cryptococcosis
2. Disseminated neoplastic disease, especially lymphosarcoma

DIAGNOSTIC AIDS

1. *Coccidioides immitis* cultured from exudate, tracheal washes, and lymph node aspirates. However, this procedure is quite hazardous (inhalation of spores may cause disease) and is not recommended
2. Direct smears of exudate or lymph node aspirates in lactophenol cotton blue or potassium hydroxide reveal thick-walled refractile spherules containing endospores
3. Two serologic tests, the complement fixation test and the precipitation test are the most widely used methods of confirming diagnosis

COMMENTS

Coccidioidomycosis is caused by a dimorphic fungus, *Coccidioides immitis*. The fungus is found in the soil in endemic areas in the southwestern United States. Chains of spores or arthrospores are the infective form and are capable of causing disease when inhaled.

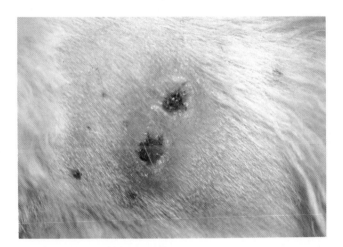

Figure 7-36 *Ulcerated, painless nodules on lateral thorax of 3-year-old mixed-breed dog from southern California. Numerous truncal cutaneous lesions were present. Patient also had generalized lymphadenopathy and was positive for* Coccidioides immitis *on serologic testing.*

Cryptococcosis

CLINICAL SIGNS

1. Cutaneous disease associated with cryptococcosis occurs only when the disease is disseminated
2. Subcutaneous nodules are the most common cutaneous sign. These nodules may ulcerate or become abscesses. They are usually multiple and, at least in the cat, involve the head most frequently
3. Ulcerations of the oral, pharyngeal, or nasal mucosa may be found
4. A firm swelling over the bridge of the nose is a common finding in the cat
5. The most common (noncutaneous) sign is a nasal discharge that may be mucopurulent, hemorrhagic, or watery. The discharge is usually chronic and may be unilateral or bilateral
6. Central nervous system involvement frequently occurs. Signs include depression, ataxia, circling, paresis, anisocoria, and blindness

DIFFERENTIAL DIAGNOSIS

1. Upper respiratory tract infection
2. Numerous other causes of varied central nervous system abnormalities
3. Other systemic mycoses
4. Neoplastic disease, especially lymphosarcoma

DIAGNOSTIC AIDS

1. Organisms are most frequently demonstrated in samples taken from cutaneous or ocular lesions and stained with India ink, methylene blue, mucicarmine, or periodic acid–Schiff. Small, round, budding yeasts surrounded by large capsule can be seen
2. Biopsies for histopathologic examination often show yeast in tissue, usually without significant tissue reaction
3. Latex agglutination to detect polysaccharide capsular antigen may be diagnostic especially in the cat

COMMENTS

Cryptococcosis is a multisystemic disease caused by the fungus *Cryptococcus neoformans*. This is a common soil fungus with worldwide distribution. The fungus exists only in the yeast form and does not have a mycelial form. The route of infection is most likely the upper respiratory tract, but this has never been proven. *Cryptococcus* is considered to be an opportunistic fungus and most frequently causes disease in immunosuppressed patients. (In man the disease is most common in patients with lymphoreticular disease and those receiving high doses of immunosuppressive drugs.)

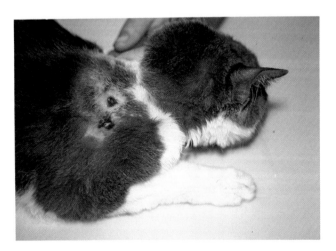

Figure 7-37   Ulcerated nodules on shoulder of 11-year-old Domestic Short-Haired cat with disseminated cryptococcosis. Patient also had oral ulcerations and nasal discharge.

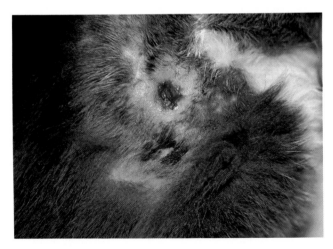

Figure 7-38   Closer view of lesions shown in Figure 7-37.

Histoplasmosis

CLINICAL SIGNS

1. The two main forms of histoplasmosis are pulmonary and intestinal. Signs include chronic cough, gradual weight loss, intermittent diarrhea, splenomegaly, hepatomegaly, fever, and anemia
2. The pulmonary and/or intestinal forms may be asymptomatic, may resolve spontaneously, or may disseminate
3. Cutaneous lesions consist of nodules that often have an ulcerated surface with draining tracts. In the cat, lesions are more common on the head and limbs

DIFFERENTIAL DIAGNOSIS

1. Other causes of respiratory and intestinal disease
2. Other systemic mycoses
3. Neoplastic disease

DIAGNOSTIC AIDS

1. Chest and abdominal radiographs to reveal characteristic abnormalities
2. Direct smears (not always diagnostic)
3. Culture of feces, bronchial washes, biopsy specimens, and bone marrow to detect *Histoplasma capsulatum* (best done by laboratory familiar with requirements of this fungus)
4. Complement fixation titers

COMMENTS

Histoplasmosis is a multisystemic disease caused by the dimorphic fungus *Histoplasma capsulatum*. It is the most common systemic mycotic disease in the dog and man in North America; the disease is less common in the cat. The fungus is found in soil in temperate and tropical climates. High numbers of organisms have been associated with soil rich in bird and bat droppings. Inhalation of the microconidia is the most common source of infection; however, ingestion is another likely source of primary infection.

Photos to illustrate this disease were not available prior to publication.

SEBACEOUS GLAND ABNORMALITIES, KERATINIZATION DEFECTS, AND NUTRITIONAL DERMATOSES

Canine seborrhea sicca

Canine seborrhea oleosa

Seborrheic dermatitis

Springer and Cocker Spaniel seborrheic disease

Vitamin A–responsive dermatosis

Canine ear margin seborrheic disease

Feline seborrheic disease

Schnauzer comedo syndrome

Idiopathic West Highland White Terrier disease (epidermal dysplasia of West Highland White Terriers, Westie "armadillo" syndrome)

Canine tail gland hyperplasia (preen gland hyperplasia)

Feline tail gland hyperplasia, (stud tail)

Feline chin acne

Callouses

Nasal hyperkeratosis

Digital hyperkeratosis

Sebaceous adenitis (granulomatous sebaceous adenitis)

Zinc dermatopathy (zinc–responsive dermatosis, zinc deficiency)

Generic dog food dermatosis

Canine Seborrhea Sicca

CLINICAL SIGNS

1. The coat is usually dull and dry
2. Fine white or gray scales are evident
3. The scales are poorly adherent to the skin surface
4. The scales may be localized or generalized
5. Odor is not usually associated with this form of seborrhea
6. Pruritus is usually mild to non-existent
7. Varying degrees of alopecia may be associated with seborrhea sicca

UNDERLYING ETIOLOGIES

1. Hypothyroidism
2. Other endocrine imbalances
3. Corticosteroid use
4. Inadequate nutrition
5. Abnormalities in intestinal absorption
6. Intestinal parasites
7. Poor grooming
8. Irritating insecticides or shampoos
9. Allergic dermatoses
10. Parasitic dermatoses
11. Pemphigus foliaceus
12. Bacterial folliculitis
13. Dermatophyte infection
14. Mycosis fungoides
15. Low environmental humidity
16. Color mutant alopecia
17. Idiopathic

DIAGNOSTIC AIDS

1. Carefully taken history
2. Complete physical and cutaneous examination
3. Appropriate tests to determine etiology; for example, skin scrapings, fungal culture, fecal floatation
4. Skin biopsies for histopathologic examination are usually not necessary and may not be diagnostic

COMMENTS

Seborrhea sicca is one of the most common and most obvious abnormalities associated with skin disease. It must be remembered that "seborrhea" is simply a clinical sign and not a diagnosis.

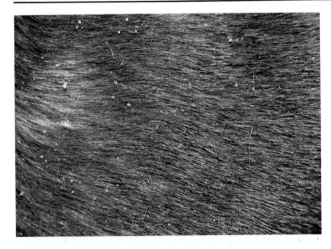

Figure 8-1   *Lateral thoracic area of hypothyroid Doberman Pinscher shows thinning of haircoat and seborrhea sicca.*

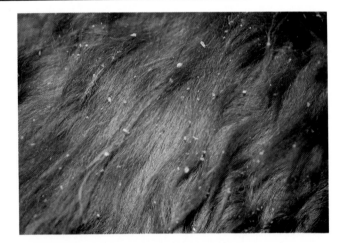

Figure 8-2   *Seborrhea sicca in patient with intestinal parasitism and flea bite hypersensitivity.*

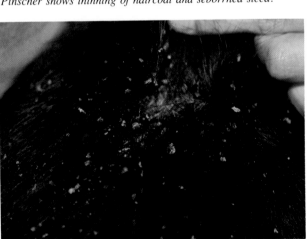

Figure 8-3   *Six-month-old mixed-breed puppy with seborrhea sicca due to* Cheyletiella *infestation.*

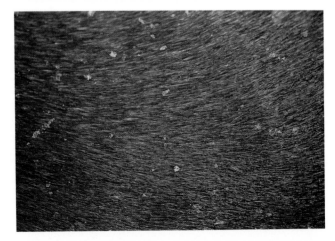

Figure 8-4   *Seborrhea sicca in young Vizsla most likely due to "too frequent" shampooing.*

Canine Seborrhea Oleosa

CLINICAL SIGNS

1. Adherent seborrheic material on the skin and hair
2. The abnormal sebaceous secretion ranges in color from white to grey to yellow and tan to brown
3. The skin and coat have a greasy feel
4. Odor is typically associated with this condition
5. The seborrhea may be localized or generalized
6. Pruritus is variable

UNDERLYING ETIOLOGIES

1. Endocrine imbalances
2. Vitamin A–responsive dermatosis
3. Zinc dermatopathy
4. Generic dog food dermatosis
5. Pemphigus foliaceus
6. Demodicosis
7. Pruritic skin diseases (allergic and parasitic)
8. Diseases resulting in chronic skin inflammation
9. Idiopathic

DIAGNOSTIC AIDS

1. Thorough cutaneous examination
2. Appropriate diagnostic tests to determine underlying etiology
3. Skin biopsies for histopathologic examination are usually helpful but may not detect underlying etiology

COMMENTS

Seborrhea oleosa is common in the dog. This condition may be a primary sebaceous gland defect or may be secondary to numerous underlying etiologies. Seborrhea oleosa is one of the most frustrating skin disorders of the dog because primary cases are usually poorly responsive to treatment and detecting the underlying etiology in secondary cases is quite difficult.

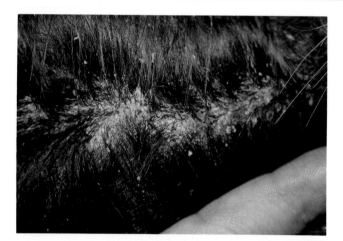

Figure 8-5 Adherent seborrheic material on back of 4-year-old mixed-breed dog. Patient was quite pruritic.

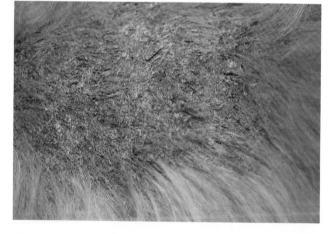

Figure 8-6 Severe, diffuse scaling and crusting on trunk of Shih Tzu with idiopathic seborrhea oleosa.

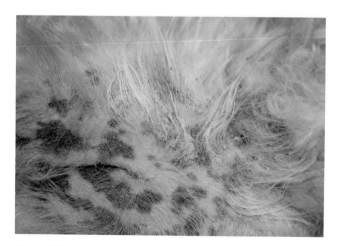

Figure 8-7 Adherent, yellow, greasy material on flank of patient with chronic inhalant allergies.

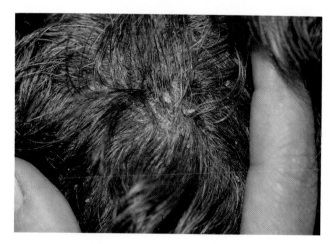

Figure 8-8 Seborrhea oleosa on shoulder of 7-year-old dog with hypothyroidism.

Seborrheic Dermatitis

CLINICAL SIGNS

1. Scaling of the skin usually with an obvious oily or greasy feeling
2. Signs of inflammation, especially erythema, are evident
3. Bacterial folliculitis is frequently a complicating factor
4. Seborrheic dermatitis may be localized or generalized
5. Pruritus is usually moderate to severe

UNDERLYING ETIOLOGIES

1. Allergic inhalant disease (atopy)
2. Flea bite hypersensitivity
3. Food hypersensitivity
4. Sarcoptic mange
5. Demodicosis
6. Endocrine imbalances
7. Zinc dermatopathy
8. Vitamin A–responsive dermatopathy
9. Idiopathic—no detectable underlying etiology

DIAGNOSTIC AIDS

1. Appropriate diagnostic tests to determine underlying etiology
2. Skin biopsies for histopathologic examination are usually diagnostic but may not detect underlying etiology

COMMENTS

Seborrheic dermatitis is a common sequela to many pruritic and inflammatory skin diseases of the dog. As with most dermatologic disorders, detection of the underlying etiology is the first step in successful treatment.

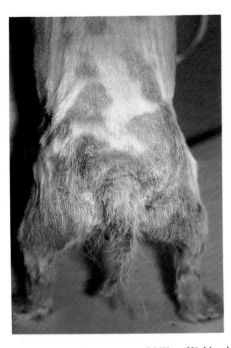

Figure 8-9 *Eleven-year-old West Highland White Terrier with patchy seborrheic dermatitis due to demodicosis.*

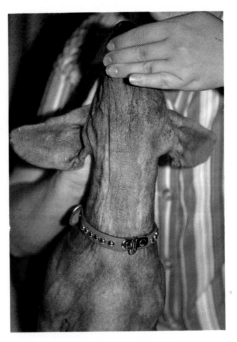

Figure 8-10 *Seborrheic dermatitis on ventral neck, chest, and ears of 5-year-old Dachshund. Patient's disease was secondary to food hypersensitivity.*

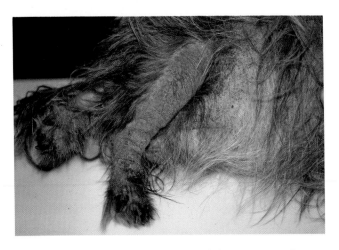

Figure 8-11   Self-induced alopecia with hyperpigmentation and seborrheic dermatitis on rear leg of Cairn Terrier with allergic inhalant disease.

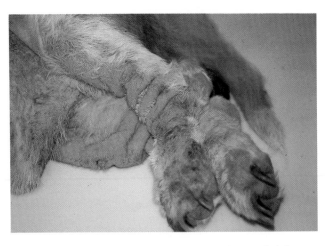

Figure 8-12   Seborrheic dermatitis on rear legs and abdomen of Beagle with severe flea bite hypersensitivity.

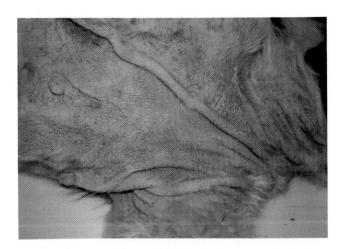

Figure 8-13   Ventral neck, axillary areas, and chest of mixed-breed dog show seborrheic dermatitis due to chronic allergic dermatitis and hypothyroidism.

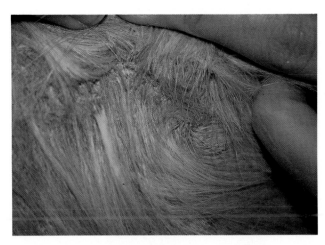

Figure 8-14   Seborrheic dermatitis on flank of Golden Retriever. Patient's disease was partially responsive to treatment for allergic inhalant disease.

Springer and Cocker Spaniel Seborrheic Disease

CLINICAL SIGNS

1. Patients have seborrhea oleosa and/or seborrheic dermatitis
2. The disease may be localized or generalized
3. The most common areas of involvement include the external ear canals, ear pinnae, ventral neck, chest, axillae, inguinal and perineal areas
4. Odor is usually associated with this disease
5. Secondary bacterial folliculitis is common
6. Patients are usually pruritic

DIFFERENTIAL DIAGNOSIS

1. Food hypersensitivity
2. Allergic inhalant disease (atopy)
3. Flea bite hypersensitivity
4. Endocrine imbalances especially hypothyroidism
5. Sarcoptic mange
6. Demodicosis
7. Dermatophyte infection
8. Zinc dermatopathy
9. Generic dog food dermatosis
10. Vitamin A–responsive dermatosis

DIAGNOSTIC AIDS

1. Appropriate diagnostic tests to rule out differentials
2. Skin biopsies for histopathologic examination are usually diagnostic

COMMENTS

Idiopathic seborrheic disease is common in Springer and Cocker Spaniels. Signs are usually evident by 18 months of age. No sex predisposition exists. Since no cause has been found for true Cocker and Springer seborrheic disease only palliative treatment is available for these unfortunate patients.

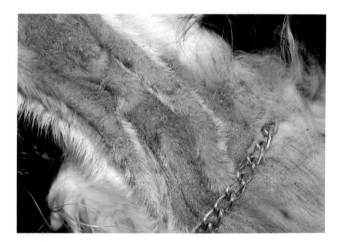

Figure 8-16　*Ventral neck of patient shown in Figure 8-15 shows seborrheic dermatitis with secondary bacterial folliculitis.*

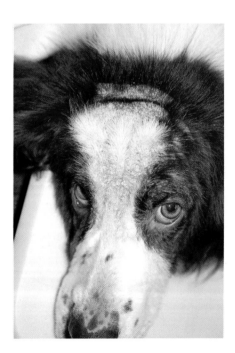

Figure 8-15　*Three-year-old male intact Springer Spaniel with seborrheic dermatitis. Patient's disease was evident by 1 year of age.*

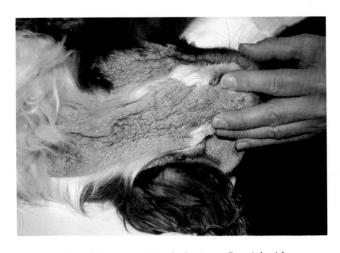

Figure 8-17 *Five-year-old male Springer Spaniel with extensive seborrheic dermatitis of chin and ventral neck.*

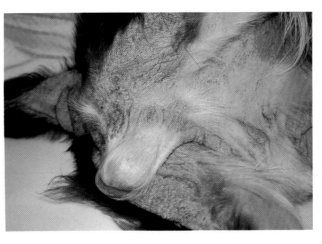

Figure 8-18 *Abdominal and inguinal areas of Springer Spaniel shown in Figure 8-17.*

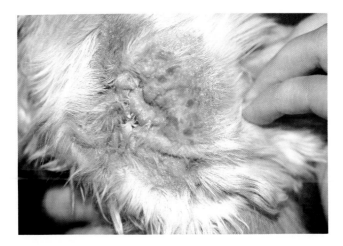

Figure 8-19 *Severe seborrheic otitis externa in young Cocker Spaniel. Patient's seborrheic disease was generalized.*

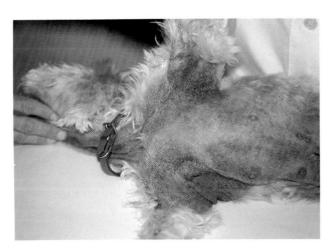

Figure 8-20 *Another view of patient shown in Figure 8-19 shows extensive hyperpigmentation and seborrheic dermatitis of ventral neck, axillary areas, and chest.*

Vitamin A–Responsive Dermatosis

CLINICAL SIGNS

1. Hyperkeratotic plaques are a hallmark of this disease
2. Follicular plugging and adherent seborrheic material may also be present
3. The most common area of involvement is the ventral chest
4. The lateral thoracic areas and abdomen may also be involved
5. Pruritus is usually mild to absent

DIFFERENTIAL DIAGNOSIS

1. Seborrhea oleosa
2. Seborrheic dermatitis
3. Springer and Cocker Spaniel seborrheic disease
4. Zinc dermatopathy
5. Generic dog food dermatosis
6. Hepatic dermatopathy
7. Sebaceous adenitis
8. Callous formation

DIAGNOSTIC AIDS

1. Skin biopsies for histopathologic examination reveal follicular orthokeratotic hyperkeratosis
2. Response to treatment with vitamin A supplements

COMMENTS

Vitamin A–responsive dermatosis is a rare disease of the dog. Cocker Spaniels may be predisposed. This condition must be differentiated from Springer and Cocker Spaniel seborrheic disease which is not vitamin A–responsive. Sebaceous adenitis may be responsive to the vitamin A derivatives but is also a separate disease entity.

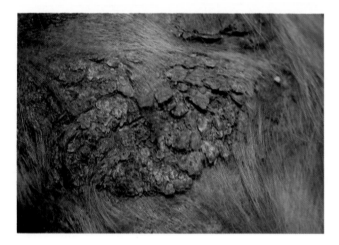

Figure 8-21   *Hyperkeratotic, vitamin A–responsive plaque on ventral chest of 4-year-old female Cocker Spaniel.*

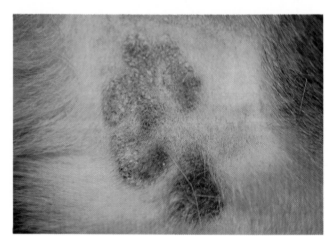

Figure 8-22   *Several hyperkeratotic plaques on chest of mixed-breed dog. Patient's seborrheic disease was responsive to vitamin A therapy.*

Canine Ear Margin Seborrheic Disease

CLINICAL SIGNS

1. Adherent seborrheic material or scales on the medial and lateral aspects of the ear pinnal margins
2. Some degree of alopecia of the pinnal margin is usually associated with this condition
3. The seborrheic disease is bilaterally symmetric
4. In severe cases the ear may become fissured
5. Patients are rarely pruritic

DIFFERENTIAL DIAGNOSIS

1. Sarcoptic mange (ear pinnae are extremely pruritic)
2. Pemphigus foliaceus
3. Flystrike
4. Frostbite

DIAGNOSTIC AIDS

1. Clinical appearance and location of lesions
2. Skin biopsies for histopathologic examination are usually helpful but the ear pinnae are difficult to biopsy

COMMENTS

Ear margin seborrheic disease is common in the dog. This condition frequently accompanies seborrhea oleosa, seborrheic dermatitis and seborrheic disease of Springer and Cocker Spaniels. It is also seen in sebaceous adenitis and zinc dermatopathy. Some cases are idiopathic.

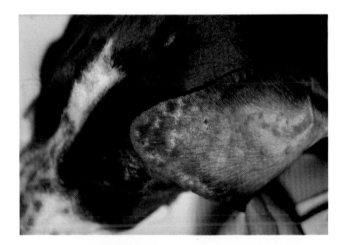

Figure 8-23 *Patchy alopecia, erythema, and scaling on medial aspect of ear pinna of male Pointer.*

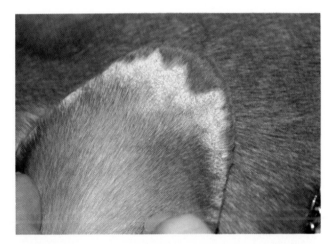

Figure 8-24 *Alopecia with adherent scales on medial aspect of pinna of Vizsla with sebaceous adenitis.*

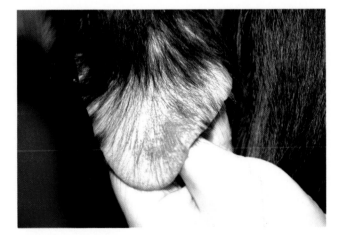

Figure 8-25 *Three-year-old Newfoundland with seborrheic disease of ear pinna.*

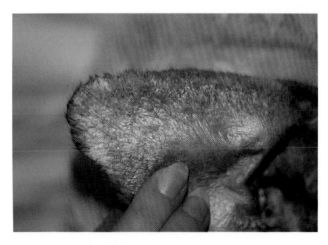

Figure 8-26 *Idiopathic ear margin seborrheic disease in young mixed German Shepherd Dog.*

Feline Seborrheic Disease

CLINICAL SIGNS

1. Most cats with "seborrhea" have fine, dry, non-adherent, white scales which resemble dandruff
2. Some patients have adherent, white to tan, scales or larger crusts
3. The disease may be generalized or localized
4. Pruritus varies depending upon the underlying etiology

UNDERLYING ETIOLOGIES

1. Low environmental humidity
2. Poor self-grooming
3. Harsh shampoos or insecticides
4. Nutritional deficiencies
5. Intestinal parasites
6. *Cheyletiella* or lice
7. Dermatophyte infection
8. Pemphigus foliaceus
9. Systemic lupus erythematosus
10. Lymphosarcoma
11. Hyperthyroidism
12. Diabetes mellitus
13. Liver disease
14. Other internal disease

DIAGNOSTIC AIDS

1. Complete physical and cutaneous examination
2. Appropriate diagnostic tests to detect underlying etiology (skin scrapings, fungal culture, skin biopsies, chemistry profile, thyroid profile)

COMMENTS

Seborrheic disease is much less common in the cat than it is in the dog. No age, breed, or sex predispositions exist. As with most skin diseases successful treatment depends upon detecting the underlying etiology.

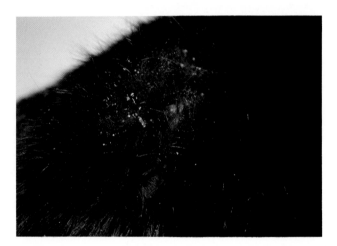

Figure 8-27   *Seborrhea sicca in 2-year-old cat due to* Cheyletiella blakei *infestation.*

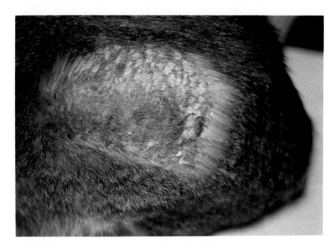

Figure 8-28   *Clumped adherent scales on back of Abyssinian cat with pemphigus foliaceus. (Hair has been clipped to visualize lesions.)*

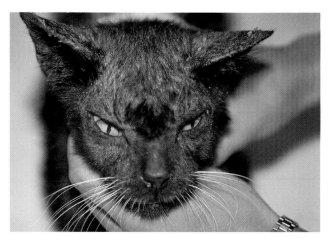

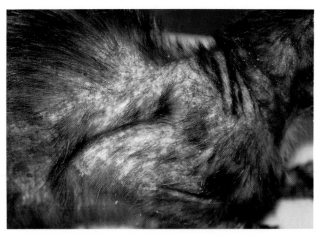

Figure 8-29   *Extensive scaling with alopecia on face and ears of 9-year old Domestic ShortHaired cat with systemic lupus erythematosus.*

Figure 8-30   *Another view of lupus patient shown in Figure 8-29.*

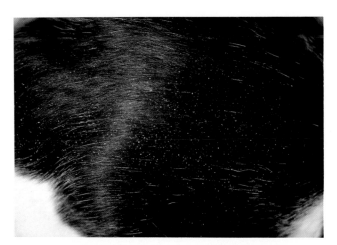

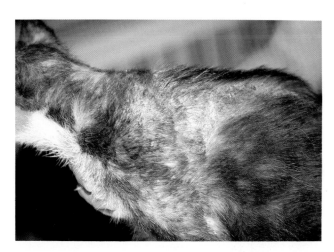

Figure 8-31   *Seborrhea sicca on trunk of mixed-breed cat caused by frequent shampooing with flea shampoo.*

Figure 8-32   *Young calico cat shows marked alopecia and scaling caused by* Microsporum canis *infection.*

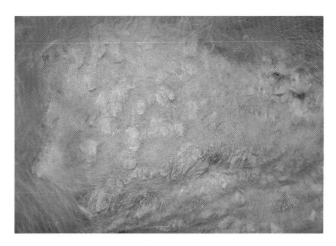

Figure 8-33   *Erythema and adherent white scales on abdomen of 14-year-old cat with cutaneous lymphosarcoma.*

Schnauzer Comedo Syndrome

CLINICAL SIGNS

1. Follicular plugging or blackhead formation along the midback
2. The disease may extend from the neck to the tail base
3. In most cases the lesions are felt by the owner before they are seen
4. Secondary bacterial folliculitis is common
5. Pruritus is minimal to absent. In cases complicated by bacterial folliculitis, pruritus may be significant

DIFFERENTIAL DIAGNOSIS

1. Bacterial folliculitis
2. Dermatophyte infection
3. Demodicosis
4. Other seborrheic disorders

DIAGNOSTIC AIDS

1. Location of lesions and breed of dog
2. Biopsies for histopathologic examination reveal dilated follicles with keratin plugs blocking the follicular opening

COMMENTS

Schnauzer comedo syndrome is relatively common. Only Miniature Schnauzers are affected; the disease has not been reported in Standard or Giant Schnauzers. There are no age or sex predispositions. Although the pathogenesis of this disease is not known, a hereditary hair follicular defect is suspected.

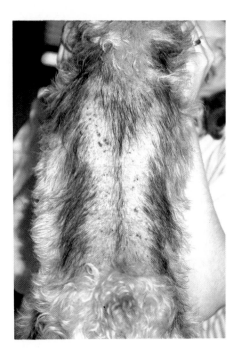

Figure 8-34   *Five-year-old Miniature Schnauzer shows self-induced alopecia and bacterial folliculitis of midback secondary to Schnauzer comedo syndrome.*

Idiopathic West Highland White Terrier Disease ("Epidermal Dysplasia" of West Highland White Terriers, Westie "Armadillo" Syndrome)

CLINICAL SIGNS

1. The earliest signs appear to be pruritus and erythema
2. Self-induced alopecia is extensive
3. Cutaneous changes secondary to chronic self-trauma include hyperpigmentation, lichenification, seborrhea oleosa, seborrheic dermatitis and bacterial folliculitis
4. The disease is usually first evident on the feet, legs, and ventrum, but it soon becomes generalized in most cases
5. Pruritus is intense

DIFFERENTIAL DIAGNOSIS

1. Sarcoptic mange
2. Food hypersensitivity
3. Allergic inhalant disease (atopy)
4. Flea bite hypersensitivity
5. Seborrheic diseases
6. Ichthyosis

DIAGNOSTIC AIDS

1. History, age, and breed of patient
2. Rule out other differentials
3. Skin biopsies for histopathologic examination may be helpful

COMMENTS

Idiopathic West Highland White Terrier skin disease is a chronic, progressive, hereditary disease of Westies. No sex predilection exists. Patients usually develop obvious signs by one year of age. Many Westies with this disease are also skin-test–positive for inhalant allergies, however, they are poorly-responsive to conventional treatment. This disease has been described as epidermal dysplasia but a true histopathologic diagnosis of epidermal dysplasia does not exist in most cases.

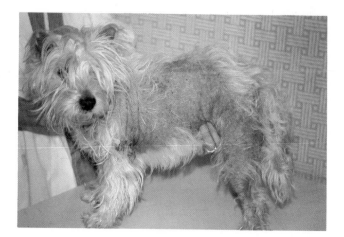

Figure 8-35　*Extensive erythema and self-induced alopecia in 18-month-old West Highland White Terrier.*

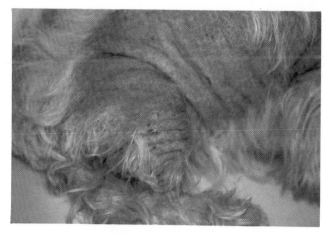

Figure 8-36　*Closer view of patient shown in Figure 8-35 shows the lichenified skin thrown into folds, hence the "armadillo" syndrome.*

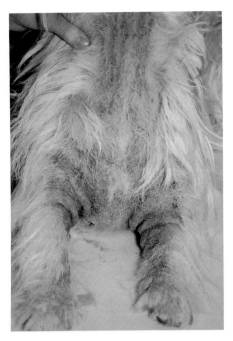

Figure 8-37   *Ventral neck, axillary areas, and chest of 3-year-old male West Highland White Terrier shows erythema, hyperpigmentation, and seborrheic changes.*

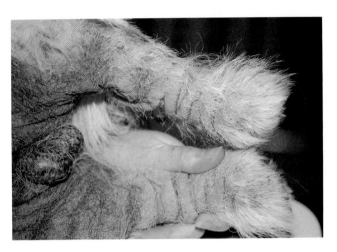

Figure 8-38   *Rear legs of Westie shown in Figure 8-37.*

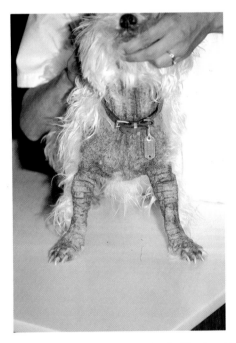

Figure 8-39   *Five-year-old male Westie with alopecia, hyperpigmentation, and lichenification. Patient's disease began at 9 months of age.*

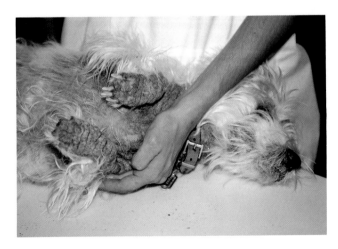

Figure 8-40   *Another view of Westie shown in Figure 8-39.*

Canine Tail Gland Hyperplasia (Preen Gland Hyperplasia)

CLINICAL SIGNS

1. Swelling of the tail gland or preen gland area which is located on the dorsum of the tail, 1 to 4 inches from the tail base
2. The involved area is round or oval in shape
3. The area may be alopecic
4. The skin may be hyperpigmented
5. Seborrheic disease is common over the tail gland
6. Secondary bacterial infection occurs in some cases
7. This condition is rarely pruritic

UNDERLYING ETIOLOGIES

1. Hypothyroidism
2. Sex hormone imbalances
3. Testicular tumors
4. Various seborrheic dermatoses

DIAGNOSTIC AIDS

1. Location of the lesion
2. Skin biopsies for histopathologic examination are rarely necessary.

COMMENTS

Tail gland hyperplasia is more common in intact male dogs. No breed predisposition has been documented. The age of affected dogs varies, but is usually greater than 4 years. The tail gland is composed of many large sebaceous glands and perianal glands which may become inflamed in patients with endocrine imbalances (especially testosterone) and seborrheic dermatoses.

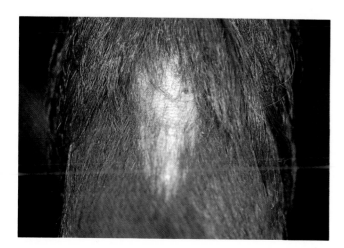

Figure 8-41   *Alopecia with a few papules involving tail gland area of Irish Setter with hypothyroidism.*

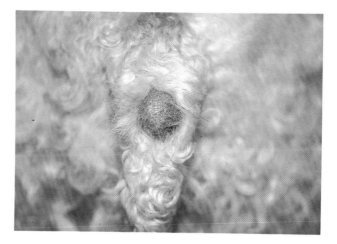

Figure 8-42   *Hyperplasia of tail gland in 11-year-old intact male Wire-haired Fox Terrier.*

Feline Tail Gland Hyperplasia (Stud Tail)

CLINICAL SIGNS

1. Inflammation of the tail gland area which lies along the entire length of the dorsum of the tail
2. The area may be partially alopecic
3. Seborrheic dermatitis is often present
4. Pruritus is minimal to absent

DIFFERENTIAL DIAGNOSIS

1. The tail gland area may become inflamed in allergic or parasitic dermatoses (especially flea bite hypersensitivity) but these diseases are not limited to the tail
2. Dermatophyte infection

DIAGNOSTIC AIDS

1. Location and appearance of the "lesion"
2. Skin biopsies for histopathologic examination are rarely necessary

COMMENTS

Tail gland hyperplasia is more common in adult male intact cats. It is also seen in neutered males and in females. The tail gland area has a high concentration of sebaceous and apocrine glands. The underlying etiology of feline tail gland hyperplasia is not known.

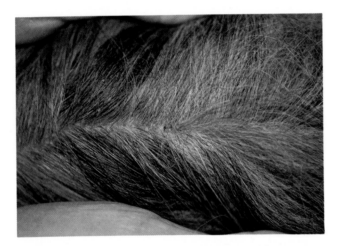

Figure 8-43   Mild tail gland hyperplasia in young female cat manifested by adherent seborrheic material and papules.

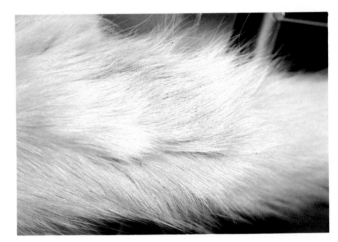

Figure 8-44   Ruffled hair, discolored by tan colored sebaceous secretion on tail of 2-year-old male intact cat.

Feline Chin Acne

CLINICAL SIGNS

1. The first sign is comedo or blackhead formation
2. The disease frequently progresses to include erythema, swelling, papules, and/or pustules
3. In some cases furunculosis and cellulitis develop
4. The chin and occasionally the lips are involved
5. This condition is rarely pruritic

DIFFERENTIAL DIAGNOSIS

1. Dermatophyte infection
2. Demodicosis

DIAGNOSTIC AIDS

1. Location and appearance of the lesions
2. Rule out other differentials by fungal culture and skin scrapings

COMMENTS

Chin acne is common in the cat. No age, breed, or sex predilections have been documented. It is thought that chin acne is caused by poor self-cleaning of the mouth and chin, or by underlying seborrheic conditions. Since the underlying etiology is not really known, treatment measures rarely cure the disease, they simply control it.

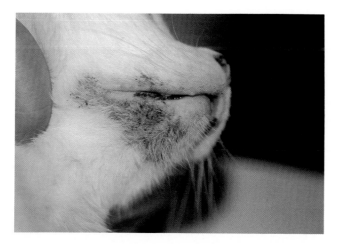

Figure 8-45 *Partial alopecia with some erythema and marked follicular plugging on chin and lips of 4-year-old male cat.*

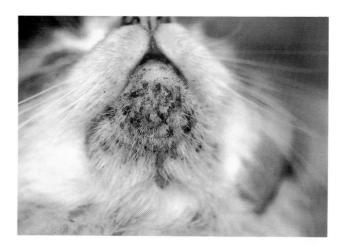

Figure 8-46 *Seven-year-old cat with chronic chin acne shows partial alopecia, erythema, swelling, and folliculitis.*

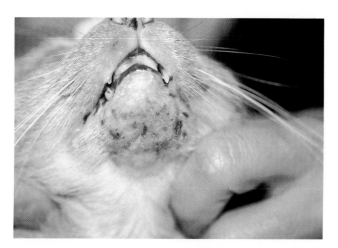

Figure 8-47 *Severe chin acne in young cat manifested by alopecia, swelling, draining tracts, and cellulitis.*

Callouses

CLINICAL SIGNS

1. Alopecia and lichenification over pressure points and boney prominences
2. The area may be erythemic or hyperpigmented
3. Secondary bacterial infection is occasionally seen
4. Callouses are usually round or oval in shape
5. Pruritus is uncommon

DIFFERENTIAL DIAGNOSES

1. Sarcoptic mange (patients may show lichenification of elbows and hocks due to pruritus)
2. Zinc dermatopathy
3. Generic dog food dermatoses

DIAGNOSTIC AIDS

1. Clinical appearance and location of lesion
2. Signalment and history

COMMENTS

Callous formation is a normal response of the skin to chronic pressure irritation. Elbow callouses are more common in the large and giant breed, short-coated dogs. Other factors contributing to callous formation are obesity and exposure to hard surfaces. The author has found that hypothyroid dogs have more severe elbow callousing than their euthyroid counterparts. Sternal callouses are most common in Dachshunds and Irish Setters. Callouses may also develop on the hocks and boney prominences of the hips. Cats rarely develop callouses.

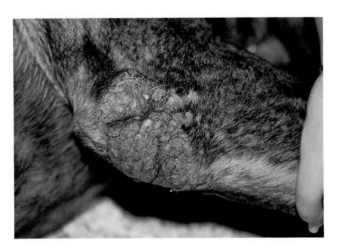

Figure 8-48 *Elbow of 18-month-old Mastiff. Patient was hypothyroid which may have contributed to excessive callous formation.*

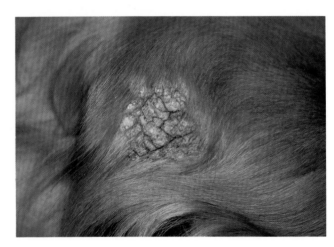

Figure 8-49 *Normal callous on elbow of 9-year-old Golden Retriever.*

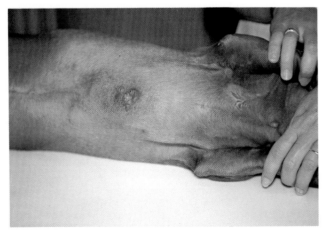

Figure 8-50 *Sternal callous in 5-year-old Standard Dachshund.*

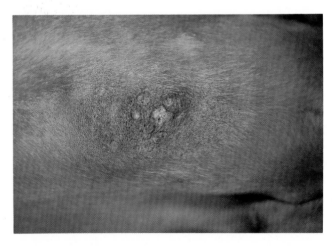

Figure 8-51 *Closer view of sternal callous shown Figure 8-50.*

Nasal Hyperkeratosis

CLINICAL SIGNS

1. Horny growths of keratin tightly adhere to the planum nasale
2. The planum nasale is extremely dry
3. Fissures and cracks may develop
4. The condition is rarely pruritic

UNDERLYING ETIOLOGIES

1. Discoid lupus erythematosus
2. Systemic lupus erythematosus
3. Pemphigus foliaceus
4. Nasal solar dermatitis
5. Zinc dermatopathy
6. Generic dog food dermatosis
7. Superficial necrolytic dermatitis
8. Canine distemper virus
9. Idiopathic

DIAGNOSTIC AIDS

1. Clinical appearance and location of lesion
2. Skin biopsies for histopathologic examination are diagnostic but usually not necessary

COMMENTS

Hyperkeratosis of the planum nasale is seen as a component of many canine skin diseases. Idiopathic nasal hyperkeratosis is most frequently seen in Cocker Spaniels and Springer Spaniels and in older dogs. This condition may be associated with digital hyperkeratosis in some patients. It is quite important to rule out the known causes of this disease before making a diagnosis of idiopathic nasal hyperkeratosis.

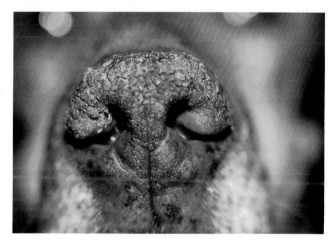

Figure 8-52   *Thirteen-year-old Vizsla with nasal hyperkeratosis shows horny keratin material tightly adherent to planum nasale.*

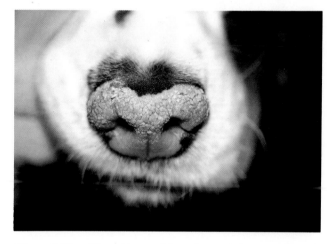

Figure 8-53   *Idiopathic nasal hyperkeratosis in young English Springer Spaniel.*

Digital Hyperkeratosis

CLINICAL SIGNS

1. Excessive keratin is present on the footpads
2. The keratin may be verrucous, ridged, or feathered
3. Cracks, deep fissures, erosions, and/or ulcers may be present
4. Pain is variable, but may be severe enough to cause lameness

UNDERLYING ETIOLOGIES

1. Pemphigus foliaceus
2. Zinc dermatopathy
3. Generic dog food dermatosis
4. Superficial necrolytic dermatitis
5. Hypothyroidism
6. Canine distemper virus
7. Idiopathic

DIAGNOSTIC AIDS

1. Location and clinical appearance of lesions
2. Skin biopsies for histopathologic examination are helpful, in some cases, to detect the underlying etiology

COMMENTS

Digital hyperkeratosis is frequently seen as a component of several canine skin diseases. The condition may be idiopathic and may be associated with nasal hyperkeratosis. Attempts to determine the underlying etiology should be made before making a diagnosis of idiopathic digital hyperkeratosis.

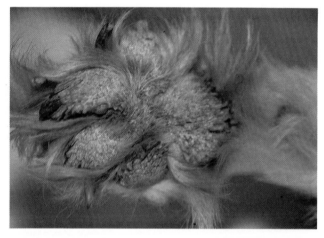

Figure 8-54 *Footpads of 8-year-old Shetland Sheepdog show digital hyperkeratosis. Patient's disease involved all four feet and was idiopathic.*

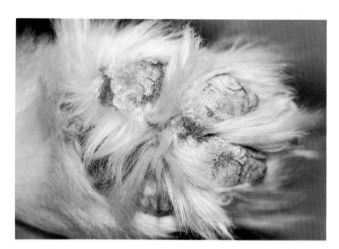

Figure 8-55 *Hyperkeratotic footpads of 3-year-old mixed Husky with zinc dermatopathy*

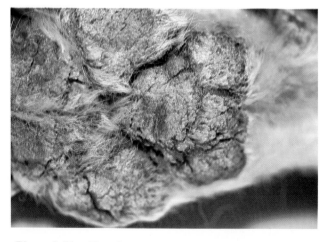

Figure 8-56 *Hyperkeratotic, cracked, and fissured footpads of 5-year-old German Shepherd Dog with pemphigus foliaceus.*

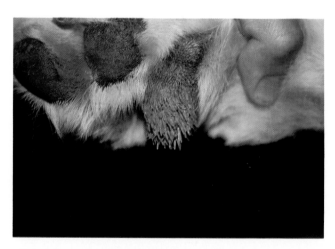

Figure 8-57 *Feathered hyperkeratosis on metacarpal pad of 4-year-old mixed-breed dog. Underlying etiology was not detected.*

Sebaceous Adenitis (Granulomatous Sebaceous Adenitis)

CLINICAL SIGNS

1. Patients have an adherent seborrheic material at the base of the hair shaft and on the skin
2. Thinning of the haircoat is a common feature
3. Remaining hair in involved areas epilates easily
4. The disease is most commonly found on the trunk, but the legs, head, and ears are frequently involved
5. Pruritus is variable

DIFFERENTIAL DIAGNOSIS

1. Dermatophyte infection
2. Demodicosis
3. Bacterial folliculitis
4. Seborrhea oleosa
5. Seborrheic dermatitis
6. Endocrine imbalances

DIAGNOSTIC AIDS

1. Appropriate diagnostic tests to rule out other differentials
2. Skin biopsies for histopathologic examination reveal hyperkeratosis and inflammation or destruction of the sebaceous glands

COMMENTS

Sebaceous adenitis is an uncommon disease of the dog. Breed predispositions include Standard Poodles, Akitas, Vizslas, and Samoyeds. No sex predisposition exists. The age at onset of clinical signs is usually between 2 and 6 years.

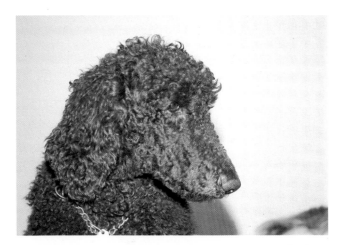

Figure 8-58 *Five-year-old female Standard Poodle with sebaceous adenitis shows mild scaling of face and shorter than normal hair on top of head.*

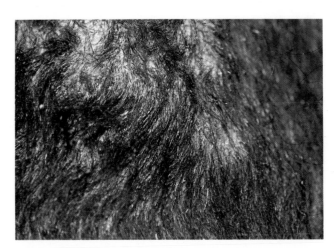

Figure 8-59 *Close-up view of shoulder of patient shown in Figure 8-58 shows marked thinning of hair and adherent seborrheic material on skin and hair.*

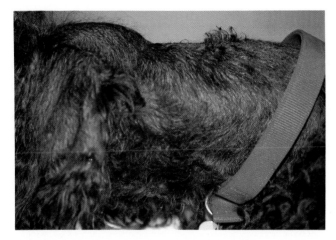

Figure 8-60 *Neck of 3-year-old male Standard Poodle with sebaceous adenitis. Patient's disease was generalized.*

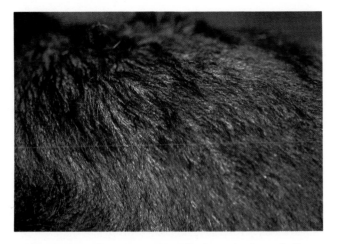

Figure 8-61 *Closer view of Poodle shown in Figure 8-60 shows thinned haircoat and adherent seborrheic scale.*

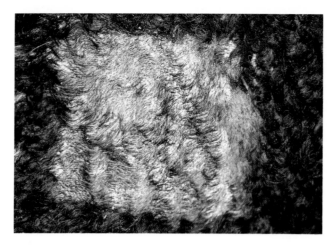

Figure 8-62   *Adherent seborrheic plaques on lateral thoracic area of Standard Poodle. Hair has been clipped to visualize lesions.*

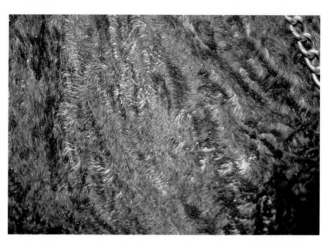

Figure 8-63   *Another Standard Poodle with sebaceous adenitis shows thinned coat and adherent seborrheic material.*

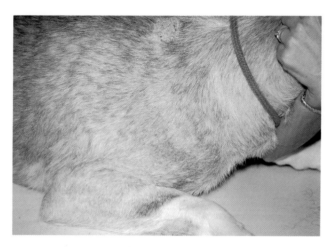

Figure 8-64   *Three-year-old male Akita with sebaceous adenitis shows moth-eaten, irregular appearance of coat.*

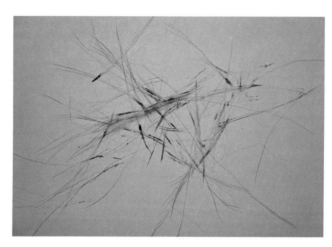

Figure 8-65   *Hairs with adherent seborrheic material from patient shown in Figure 8-64. Hairs were easily epilated.*

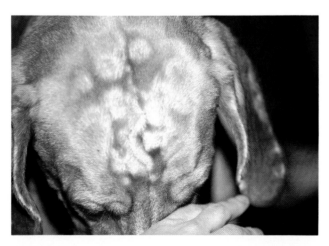

Figure 8-66   *Circular, coalescing areas of alopecia and scaling on head of young Vizsla with sebaceous adenitis. Ear pinnae are also involved.*

Zinc Dermatopathy (Zinc–Responsive Dermatosis, Zinc Deficiency)

CLINICAL SIGNS

1. Skin changes include alopecia, erythema, scaling, and crusting
2. The most common areas of involvement are the face and ears
3. The elbows, hocks, and other pressure points may be affected
4. Hyperkeratosis of the footpads is often a feature
5. Alopecia, scaling, and hyperpigmentation of the scrotum, vulva, and surrounding areas may be seen
6. Patients are usually not pruritic

DIFFERENTIAL DIAGNOSIS

1. Demodicosis
2. Dermatophyte infection
3. Pemphigus foliaceus
4. Generic dog food dermatosis
5. Hepatic dermatopathy

DIAGNOSTIC AIDS

1. Thorough history and clinical signs
2. Appropriate diagnostic tests to rule out differentials
3. Skin biopsies for histopathologic examination reveal marked follicular and diffuse parakeratotic hyperkeratosis

COMMENTS

Zinc dermatopathy is a common disease of the dog and is seen most frequently in Siberian Huskies and Alaskan Malamutes. These breeds may have a genetic defect resulting in decreased zinc absorption from the intestines. The disease is also seen in rapidly growing, large breed puppies that are fed a diet high in cereals or a diet that is oversupplemented with minerals, especially calcium.

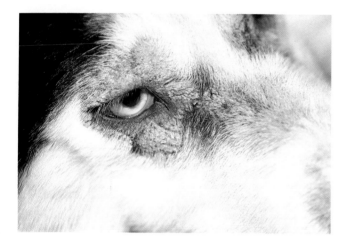

Figure 8-67 *Eighteen-month-old Siberian Husky shows alopecia and thick scales involving periocular area and extending down bridge of nose.*

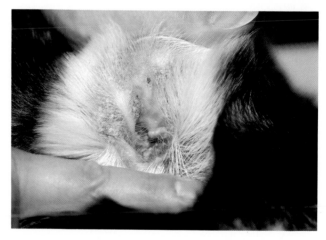

Figure 8-68 *Scaling and erythema on medial aspect of ear pinna of Husky shown in Figure 8-67.*

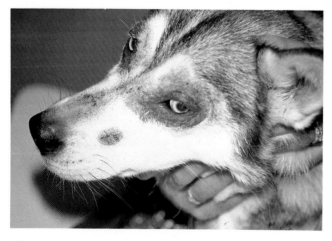

Figure 8-69 *Alopecia, erythema, hyperpigmentation, and scaling on face of 4-year-old Siberian Husky.*

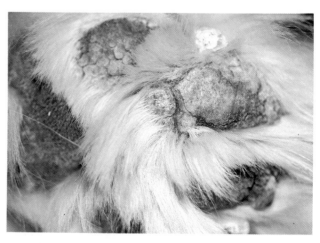

Figure 8-70 *Hyperkeratotic, fissured footpads of 3-year-old Husky with zinc dermatopathy.*

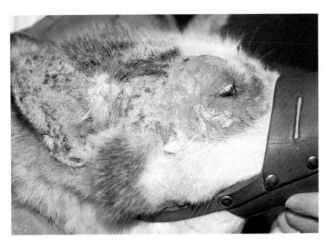

Figure 8-71 *Severe alopecia, erythema, and scaling with some ulceration on face and ear pinna of middle-aged Husky.*

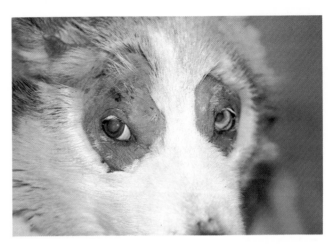

Figure 8-72 *Patient shown in Figure 8-71 after 6 weeks of zinc supplementation.*

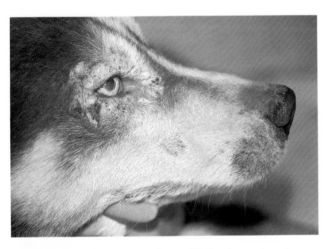

Figure 8-73 *Six-year-old Siberian Husky shows alopecia, crusting, and ulceration of periocular area. Muzzle is also involved in this case of zinc dermatopathy.*

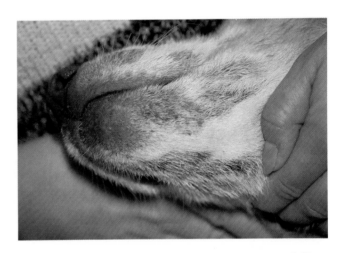

Figure 8-74 *Another view of patient shown in Figure 8-73.*

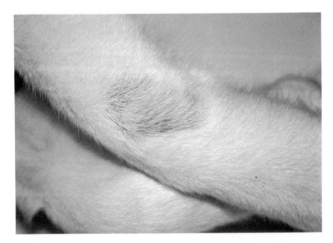

Figure 8-75 *Patch of alopecia and erythema with mild scaling over carpal area of 6-year-old Siberian Husky with zinc dermatopathy.*

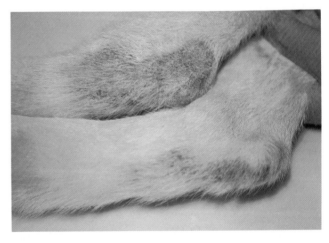

Figure 8-76 *Erythematous, scaling hocks of patient shown in Figure 8-75.*

Generic Dog Food Dermatosis

CLINICAL SIGNS

1. The most common lesions are extensive crusting, and scaling
2. Alopecia and papules are frequently seen
3. Severe cases have erosions and ulcerations
4. Lesions are usually bilaterally symmetric
5. Areas of involvement include the face, pressure points, distal extremities, footpads, and mucocutaneous junctions
6. Patients may be lethargic, depressed, and febrile
7. Generalized peripheral lymphadenopathy may be present
8. Pitting edema of the limbs has been reported
9. Most patients are not pruritic

DIFFERENTIAL DIAGNOSIS

1. Zinc dermatopathy
2. Seborrheic disease
3. Pemphigus foliaceus/vegetans
4. Systemic lupus erythematosus
5. Demodicosis
6. Dermatophyte infection
7. Bacterial dermatitis

DIAGNOSTIC AIDS

1. History of patient eating a "generic" dog food which does not meet the National Research Council's (NRC) recommendations
2. Skin biopsies for histopathological examination show superficial perivascular dermatitis with diffuse parakeratotic hyperkeratosis

COMMENTS

Generic dog food dermatosis has recently been reported. Young dogs appear to be predisposed. Clinical signs develop several weeks after starting the suspect diet which may contain proteins mainly of plant origin. These diets which do not meet the NRC recommendations for balanced nutrition are often high in phytates which lower the absorption of dietary minerals. Generic dog food dermatosis most likely is caused by severe zinc deficiency or multiple mineral deficiency.

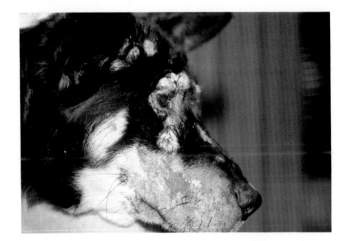

Figure 8-77   *Nine-month-old mixed-breed dog shows patchy areas of alopecia, erythema, and scaling on face.*

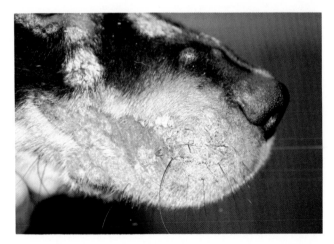

Figure 8-78   *Closer view of patient shown in Figure 8-77.*

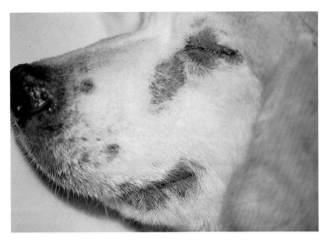

Figure 8-79 *Moist dermatitis manifested by alopecia, erythema, and oozing on face of young mixed-breed dog fed a multi-mineral deficient diet.*

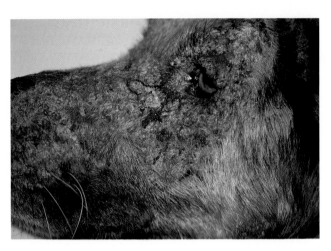

Figure 8-80 *Extensive alopecia, crusting, and fissuring on face of 6-year-old German Shepherd Dog fed an unbalanced "vegetarian" diet.*

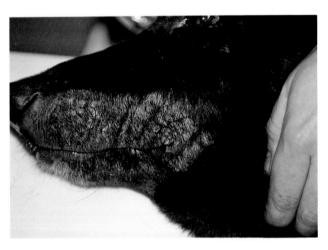

Figure 8-81 *Mixed German Shepherd Dog shows crusting and inflammation of muzzle. (Hair has been clipped to visualize lesions.)*

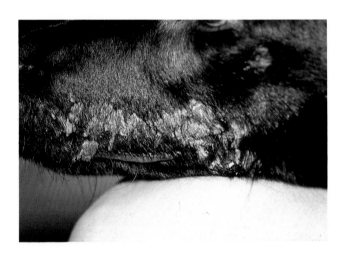

Figure 8-82 *Chocolate Labrador Retriever with crusted facial lesions apparently caused by "generic" dog food.*

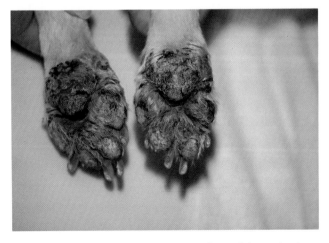

Figure 8-83 *Swollen, hyperkeratotic, fissured footpads of young mixed-breed dog with generic dog food dermatosis.*

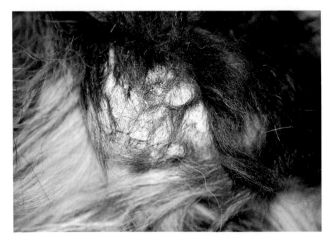

Figure 8-84 *Extensive crusting and scaling on elbow of mixed-breed Collie. Patient also had facial and footpad lesions.*

CONGENITAL AND HEREDITARY DERMATOSES

Acral mutilation syndrome

Black hair follicular dysplasia

Canine alopecia universalis (Chinese Crested Dog)

Canine ichthyosis (fish scale disease)

Color mutant alopecia

Congenital alopecia

Cutaneous aesthenia (Ehlers-Danlos syndrome, rubber puppy syndrome)

Dermatomyositis (Sheltie/Collie syndrome, formerly called epidermolysis bullosa)

Dermoid sinus

Feline alopecia universalis (Sphinx cat)

Feline hypotrichosis (Devon Rex)

Hypotrichosis of Irish Water Spaniels

Pattern baldness of Dachshunds

Acral Mutilation Syndrome

CLINICAL SIGNS

1. One of the earliest signs is licking and biting of all four feet, especially the rear feet. This eventually leads to self-mutilation
2. The feet and toes become swollen
3. There is a total loss of temperature in the feet
4. Since there is also loss of pain sensation, affected pups may actually chew off their toes and continue to walk, without any discomfort

DIFFERENTIAL DIAGNOSIS

1. Frostbite
2. Autoimmune disorders

DIAGNOSTIC AIDS

1. Clinical signs as well as age and breed of patient
2. Skin biopsies for histopathologic examination of nerve tissue at necropsy

COMMENTS

Acral mutilation syndrome is a very rare sensory neuropathy that has been reported in English Pointers and German Short-Haired Pointers. Clinical signs are apparent between 3 and 5 months of age. The mode of inheritance is probably autosomal recessive.

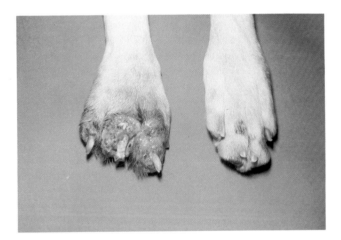

Figure 9-1 Severe self-induced ulceration and mutilation on right forefoot of English Pointer pup. (Slide courtesy of Dr. John M. MacDonald, Auburn, Alabama.)

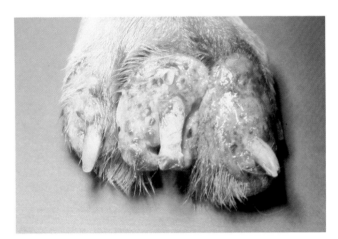

Figure 9-2 Closer view of patient shown in Figure 9-1. (Slide courtesy of Dr. John M. MacDonald, Auburn, Alabama.)

Black Hair Follicular Dysplasia

CLINICAL SIGNS

1. Sparse, abnormal hair on black portions of the coat
2. The hair in involved areas is usually brittle and broken and lacks the normal shine
3. Seborrhea sicca may be present in black haired areas
4. The other colored (white, tan) portions of the coat are normal
5. Patients are nonpruritic

DIFFERENTIAL DIAGNOSIS

1. Endocrine alopecias that may, by coincidence, involve only the black coat portions
2. Demodicosis
3. Dermatophyte infection
4. Color mutant alopecias

DIAGNOSTIC AIDS

1. Distribution of abnormal hair coat
2. Abnormality present at birth
3. Skin biopsies for histopathologic examination show distortions of hair follicular walls and follicular plugging of involved black hairs

COMMENTS

Black hair follicular dysplasia is a rare dermatologic disorder that has been reported in several breeds including mongrels, Dachshunds, Bearded Collies, Papillons, and Schipperkes. The mode of inheritance is not known.

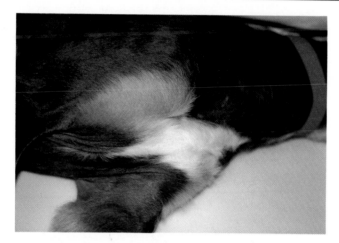

Figure 9-3 *Chest area of 5-month-old Saluki shows normal tan and white hairs. The black coat, however, is shorter and sparser than normal.*

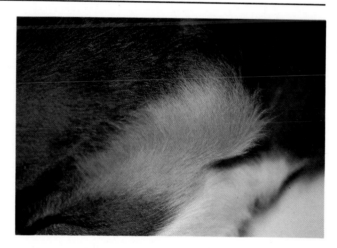

Figure 9-4 *Closer view of Salukis' haircoat shown in Figure 9-3.*

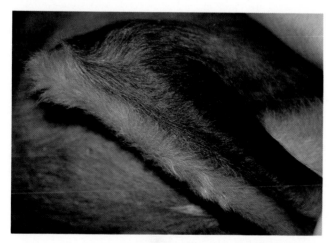

Figure 9-5 *Right foreleg of patient shown in Figures 9-3 and 9-4. Tan hair is normal and black hair is short, brittle, and sparse.*

Canine Alopecia Universalis (Chinese Crested Dog)

CLINICAL SIGNS

1. Near-total alopecia of the body, tail, and legs
2. A crest of hair of varying thickness and size is present on the head
3. Some hair may be present on the face and head. Hair on the head is a desirable trait
4. The tail may be partially haired
5. The color of the alopecic skin varies, but it usually is a grey-blue color because of the presence of extensive follicular plugging or blackhead formation

DIFFERENTIAL DIAGNOSIS

1. Various endocrine imbalances
2. Demodicosis
3. Dermatophyte infection

COMMENTS

There are two varieties of the Chinese Crested dog, the Hairless and the Powderpuff. The Hairless variety has the signs described above. The Powderpuff has a normal-appearing coat. Severely abnormal dentition frequently accompanies the hairlessness. Other "hairless" breeds include the Mexican Hairless Dog, Xoloitzcuintl, Peruvian Hairless Dog, Abyssinian Dog, African Sand Dog, and Turkish Naked Dog.

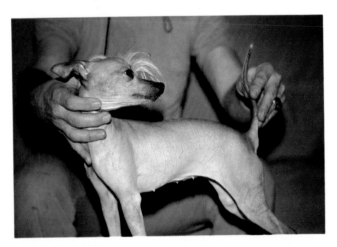

Figure 9-6 *One-year-old female Chinese Crested Dog shows total alopecia except for few hairs on head.*

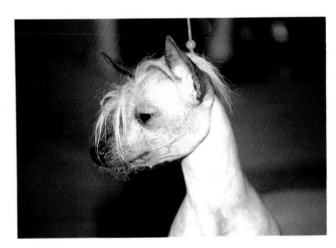

Figure 9-7 *Closer view of hairless dog shown in Figure 9-6.*

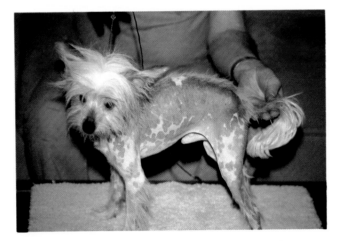

Figure 9-8 *Three-year-old male Chinese Crested Dog. Hair on this animal's head and tail is desirable; body hair is an undesirable trait.*

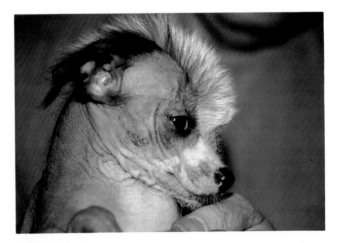

Figure 9-9 *Two-month-old Chinese Crested pup shows skin pigmentation and "mohawk" on head.*

Canine Ichthyosis (Fish Scale Disease)

CLINICAL SIGNS

1. Tightly adhering, fine white scales cover most of the body
2. Sticky, adherent brownish flakes are found on skin and haircoat
3. Varying degrees of digital hyperkeratosis may be present
4. Pruritus varies from nonexistent to moderate

DIFFERENTIAL DIAGNOSIS

1. Zinc dermatopathy
2. Nasodigital hyperkeratosis
3. Various seborrheic dermatoses
4. Sebaceous adenitis

DIAGNOSTIC AIDS

1. Presence of disease at birth
2. Breed of dog may be helpful
3. Generalized distribution of disease
4. Skin biopsies for histopathologic examination show orthokeratotic hyperkeratosis, granulosis, and mitotic figures in keratinocytes

COMMENTS

Ichthyosis is a rare congenital disease of dogs. West Highland White Terriers may be predisposed. Females may be predisposed. The mode(s) of inheritance of canine ichthyosis has not been documented. Since there are several types of congenital ichthyoses in the dog, the clinical signs may vary greatly. Therefore diagnosis must be based on histopathologic examination of biopsy specimens and not on the clinical appearance.

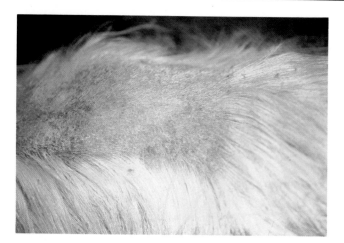

Figure 9-10   *Tightly adherent white and tan scales on midback of 4-year-old female West Highland White Terrier. (Hair has been shaved from involved area.)*

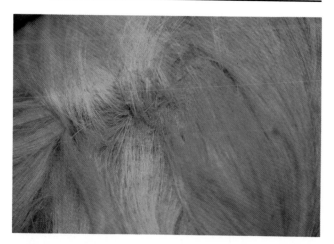

Figure 9-11   *Another truncal view of patient shown in Figure 9-10.*

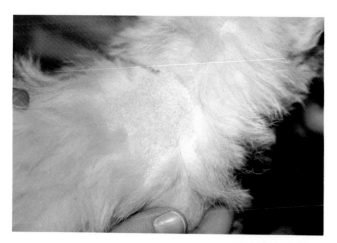

Figure 9-12   *Lamellar ichthyosis in a 5-week-old West Highland White Terrier. This pup is daughter of patient shown in Figures 9-10 and 9-11. (Hair has been shaved from involved area.)*

Color Mutant Alopecia

CLINICAL SIGNS

1. Thinning of the blue- or fawn-colored haircoat with brittle, broken, stubbly hairs
2. Scaling of skin in blue or fawn areas
3. The hair and skin in tan or white areas is normal
4. Blackhead formation and folliculitis are common secondary complications

DIFFERENTIAL DIAGNOSIS

1. Demodicosis
2. Hypothyroidism
3. Other endocrine imbalances
4. Other causes of seborrheic dermatoses
5. Dermatophyte infection

DIAGNOSTIC AIDS

1. Breed of dog and coat color are quite helpful
2. Distribution of alopecic pattern and abnormal skin
3. Skin biopsies for histopathologic examination may be helpful but not diagnostic

COMMENTS

Color mutant alopecia is seen most commonly in blue and fawn Doberman Pinschers. The author has also seen the abnormality in fawn Irish Setters, blue and fawn Dachshunds, blue Great Danes, blue Newfoundlands, and blue mixed-breed dogs. The condition has also been reported in blue-colored dogs of the following breeds: Italian Greyhounds, Whippets, Chow Chows, and Standard Poodles. No sex predilection has been reported. The patient may have a normal haircoat at birth and through puppyhood and develop the alopecic pattern later in life.

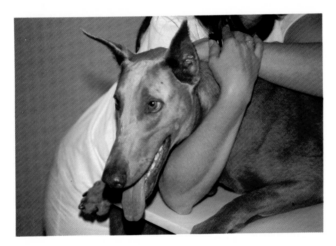

Figure 9-13 *Fawn-colored Doberman Pinscher. Thickness of coat on face, shoulders, and legs is relatively normal.*

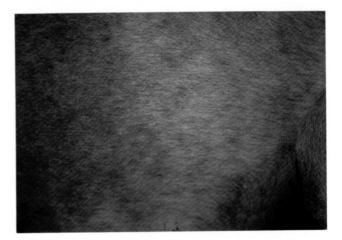

Figure 9-14 *Close-up view of lateral thoracic area of patient shown in Figure 9-13. Note sparseness of coat.*

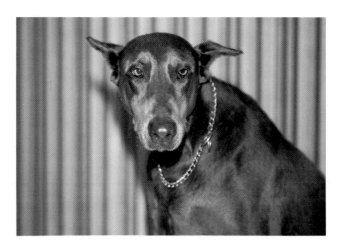

Figure 9-15 *Blue and tan Doberman Pinscher. From this view patient's coat appears quite normal.*

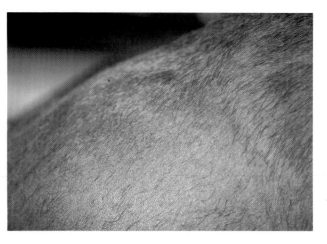

Figure 9-16 *Close-up photograph of truncal coat of patient shown in Figure 9-15. Coat is extremely sparse and coarse.*

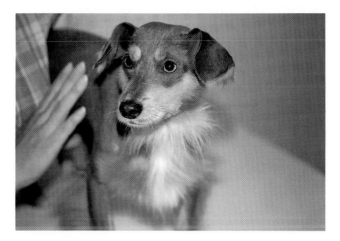

Figure 9-17 *Three-year-old mixed-breed dog with blue-color mutant alopecia. The white and tan-colored haircoat is normal.*

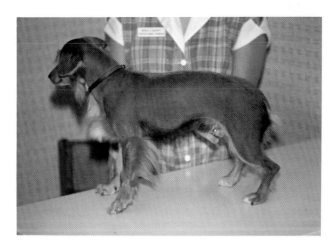

Figure 9-18 *Another view of patient shown in Figure 9-17.*

Congenital Alopecia

CLINICAL SIGNS

1. Bilaterally symmetric alopecia involving various areas of the body
2. Alopecic skin may also lack sebaceous glands and sweat glands
3. Affected dogs are nonpruritic

DIFFERENTIAL DIAGNOSIS

1. Various endocrine imbalances
2. Black hair follicular dysplasia
3. Demodicosis
4. Dermatophyte infection

DIAGNOSTIC AIDS

1. Unusual alopecic pattern
2. Alopecia present at birth
3. Skin biopsies for histopathologic examination show complete absence of hair follicles, sebaceous glands, and apocrine glands

COMMENTS

Congenital alopecia is a rare disease of the dog. The condition has been reported in Poodles and Belgian Shepherds. Males appear to be predisposed. The mode of inheritance has not been documented.

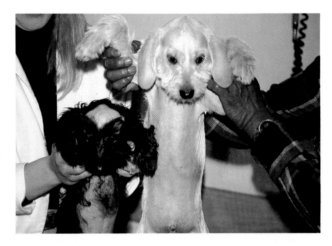

Figure 9-19 *Littermate male mixed-breed Poodle puppies with obvious alopecia involving head and ventrum.*

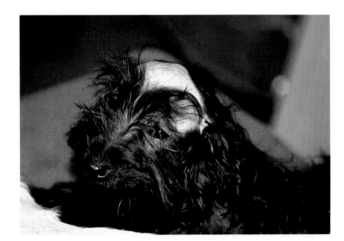

Figure 9-20 *Closer view of one of puppies with congenital alopecia shown in Figure 9-19.*

Cutaneous Aesthenia (Ehlers-Danlos Syndrome, Rubber Puppy Syndrome)

CLINICAL SIGNS

1. Hyperextensible, easily stretched skin
2. The skin is fragile and tears easily, especially with minimal self-trauma, such as scratching
3. The tears usually heal quickly, leaving scars
4. Joint laxity is seen in some patients

DIFFERENTIAL DIAGNOSIS

1. Thin, fragile skin is often seen in patients with hyperadrenocorticism
2. Some breeds such as Bloodhound and Basset Hound normally have hyperextensible skin

DIAGNOSTIC AIDS

1. A diagnosis often can be made based upon the classic clinical signs
2. Skin biopsies for histopathologic examination may show shortened, fragmented, and disoriented collagen fibers

COMMENTS

Cutaneous aesthenia is an uncommon disease in the dog and cat. No breed or sex predispositions have been documented. The disease is usually diagnosed in young animals. The mode of inheritance is a simple dominant autosomal trait. Defects in collagen fibrillogenesis are responsible for the abnormal physical properties of affected skin.

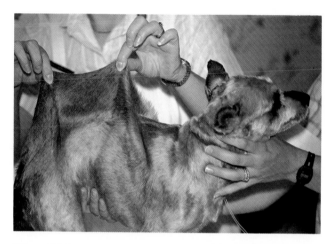

Figure 9-21 Hyperextensible skin in 4-year-old female Miniature Schnauzer.

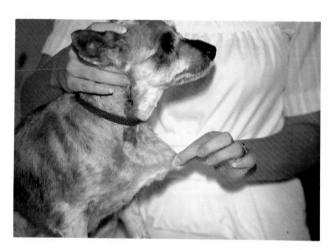

Figure 9-22 Another demonstration of hyperextensible skin of patient shown in Figure 9-21.

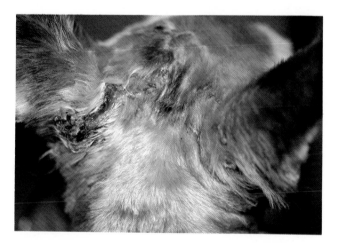

Figure 9-23 Multiple cutaneous tears on head of patient shown in Figures 9-21 and 9-22. These tears were result of scratching caused by allergic inhalant disease.

Dermatomyositis (Sheltie/Collie Syndrome, formerly called epidermolysis bullosa)

CLINICAL SIGNS

1. Skin changes include alopecia, erythema, scales, crusts, blisters, erosions, ulcerations, and scarring
2. Hypopigmentation and depigmentation may accompany these changes
3. The most common areas of involvement are the face, ear pinnae, bony prominences of the limbs, and tail
4. Muscle atrophy may be quite evident, especially involving the temporal muscles
5. Some severely affected patients are weak and dysphagic due to extensive muscle degeneration
6. Patients are usually nonpruritic and nonpainful

DIFFERENTIAL DIAGNOSIS

1. Discoid lupus erythematosus
2. Pemphigus erythematosus
3. Demodicosis
4. Dermatophyte infection
5. Nasal solar dermatitis
6. Bacterial skin infection

DIAGNOSTIC AIDS

1. Age and breed of patient as well as the location of lesions
2. Skin and muscle biopsies for histopathologic examination are usually diagnostic
3. Biopsies for direct immunofluorescence testing may be positive
4. Antinuclear antibody tests are negative
5. Electromyelogram studies

COMMENTS

Dermatomyositis is a hereditary, idiopathic, systemic, inflammatory connective tissue disorder which primarily affects Shetland Sheepdogs, Collies, and their crosses. Signs are evident between 1 and 6 months of age. No sex predilection has been reported. Signs may vary from mild cutaneous disease to severe muscle involvement and death. Although the pathomechanism of this disease in the dog is unknown, immune complex deposition may play a role.

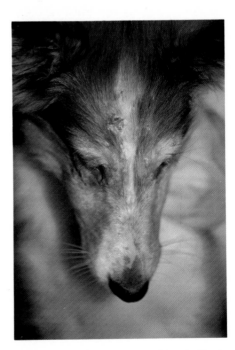

Figure 9-24 *Three-month-old male Shetland Sheepdog with dermatomyositis. Note patchy alopecia, erythema, scales, and crusts.*

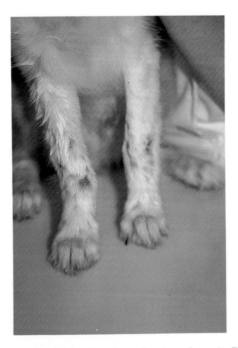

Figure 9-25 *Forelegs of patient shown in Figure 9-24. Alopecia, erythema, and erosions are seen.*

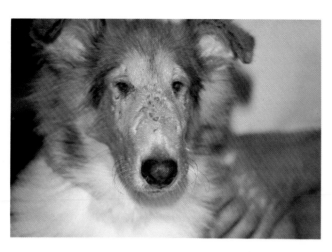

Figure 9-26 *Five-month-old male Collie with dermatomyositis. Patchy alopecia with hyperpigmentation and some areas of erythema are seen.*

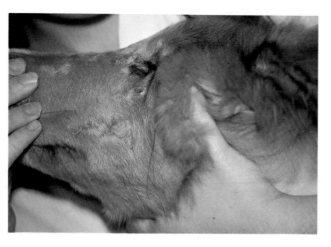

Figure 9-27 *Another view of Collie pup shown in Figure 9-26.*

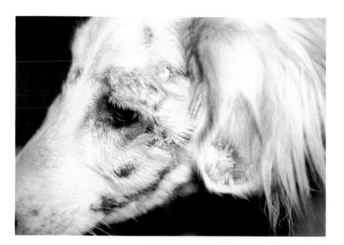

Figure 9-28 *Nine-month-old mixed Shetland Sheepdog shows dermatomyositis lesions on face and ear pinnae.*

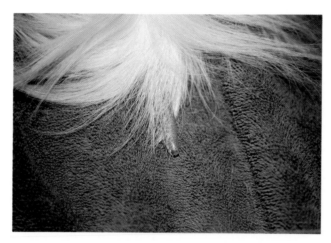

Figure 9-29 *Alopecia and erythema on tail tip of patient shown in Figure 9-28.*

Dermoid Sinus

CLINICAL SIGNS

1. Swellings or cysts on the dorsal midline which may open and drain periodically
2. A tuft of hair often protrudes from the skin opening
3. Lesions may occur anywhere along the dorsal midline but are most frequently found in the cervical area
4. If the sinus becomes infected or communicates with the dura mater, neurologic signs usually occur

DIFFERENTIAL DIAGNOSIS

1. Deep bacterial or fungal infections
2. Fight wounds
3. Other "cystic" structures (sebaceous cysts, keratoacanthomas) along the dorsal midline

DIAGNOSTIC AIDS

1. Clinical appearance, location of lesion(s), and breed of dog are quite helpful
2. Skin biopsies for histopathologic examination are usually diagnostic

COMMENTS

Dermoid sinuses are congenital defects caused by incomplete separation of the spinal cord and the skin from the ectodermal layer during embryonic development. They are most commonly found in the Rhodesian Ridgeback; however, they have also been reported in other breeds of dogs. The exact mode of inheritance is unknown, but it is thought to be a simple recessive trait.

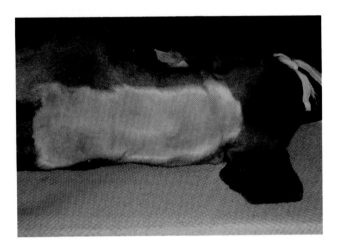

Figure 9-30 *Dermoid sinus swelling is evident in cervical area of young male Rhodesian Ridgeback. Hair in involved area has been shaved. (Slide courtesy of Dr. Diane E. Bevier, Boston, Massachusetts.)*

Feline Alopecia Universalis (Sphinx Cat)

CLINICAL SIGNS

1. The body is covered by a very short down that is almost imperceptible to both the eye and touch
2. The skin has the feel of suede
3. The skin has a wrinkled appearance that is more pronounced in kittens
4. Whiskers and eyebrows may be present
5. Short, tightly packed hair may be present on the ears, muzzle, tail, feet, and scrotum
6. Heterozygous Sphinx cats have more down on the body than have homozygous individuals
7. An excessive production of sebum from the sebaceous glands results in a brownish, greasy buildup on the skin
8. A copius amount of brown-black cerumen is almost always present in the external ear canals

DIFFERENTIAL DIAGNOSIS

1. Self-induced alopecia
2. Feline endocrine alopecia

COMMENTS

The Sphinx cat is an extremely rare breed. It is estimated that fewer than 100 Sphinx cats exist in the world. The Sphinx is often bred to the Devon Rex to produce kittens that are Sphinx, Devon Rex, or normal haired.

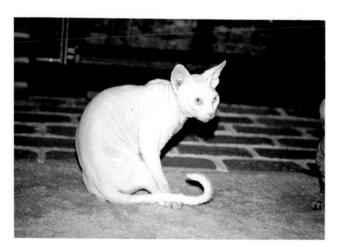

Figure 9-31 *Four-year-old male Sphinx cat shows near-total alopecia except for tail.*

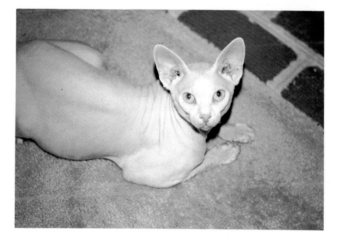

Figure 9-32 *Another view of Sphinx cat shown in Figure 9-31.*

Feline Hypotrichosis (Devon Rex)

CLINICAL SIGNS

1. Alopecia may involve any part of the body
2. In the Devon Rex the alopecia primarily involves the ventral neck, chest, and abdomen
3. The alopecic pattern is bilaterally symmetric
4. Skin in alopecic areas appears normal

DIFFERENTIAL DIAGNOSIS

1. Self-induced alopecia
2. Feline endocrine alopecia

COMMENTS

Feline hypotrichosis has been reported in the Devon Rex cat and in the Siamese cat. The condition is an autosomal recessive trait.

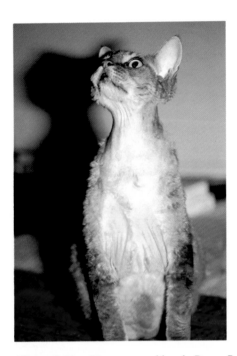

Figure 9-33 *Eleven-year-old male Devon Rex cat shows significant alopecia of ventral neck, chest, and abdomen.*

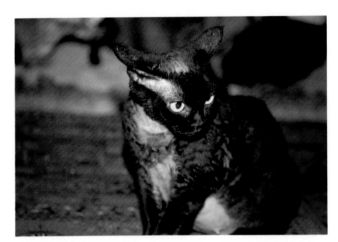

Figure 9-34 *Alopecia of head, neck, chest, and abdomen in six-year-old female Devon Rex cat.*

Hypotrichosis of Irish Water Spaniels

CLINICAL SIGNS

1. Alopecia may involve the ventral neck, rump, perineum, caudal thighs, and/or tail
2. The skin in alopecic areas usually appears normal but may be dry and scaly
3. Patients are not pruritic

DIFFERENTIAL DIAGNOSIS

1. Hypothyroidism
2. Testosterone–responsive alopecia
3. Estrogen–responsive alopecia

DIAGNOSTIC AIDS

1. Breed of dog and alopecic pattern
2. Rule out other differentials

COMMENTS

Hypotrichosis of Irish Water Spaniels is a hereditary pattern baldness. The mode of inheritance is not known. No sex predisposition has been documented. The alopecic pattern is noticeable by 2 years of age.

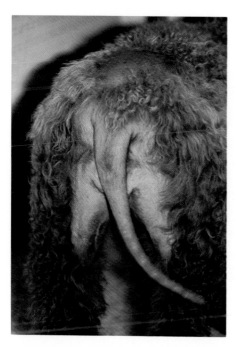

Figure 9-35   Caudal view of 3-year-old female intact Irish Water Spaniel shows alopecia of rump, perineum, tail, and caudal thighs.

Pattern Baldness of Dachshunds

CLINICAL SIGNS

1. Female Dachshunds have alopecia mainly involving the ventral neck, chest, and abdominal areas, Alopecia may be present in other areas
2. The alopecia in male Dachshunds usually involves the ear pinnae; however, other areas may be involved
3. Patients are not pruritic
4. The skin in alopecic areas may be leathery and hyperpigmented

DIFFERENTIAL DIAGNOSIS

1. Hypothyroidism
2. Estrogen–responsive dermatoses
3. Testosterone–responsive dermatoses
4. Hyperadrenocorticism

DIAGNOSTIC AIDS

1. Breed of patient and distribution of alopecia
2. Rule out other differentials

COMMENTS

Pattern baldness of Dachshunds is a hereditary disorder which most frequently involves Short-Haired Miniature and Standard Dachshunds but may also involve Long-Haired and Wire-Haired Dachshunds. There is no sex predisposition. The alopecic pattern is usually noticeable by 1 year of age and in most cases becomes gradually more severe as the patient ages.

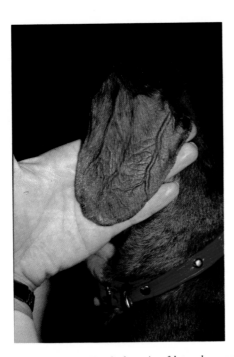

Figure 9-36 *Total alopecia of lateral aspect of ear pinna of 4-year-old male Dachshund. Patient's alopecia involved only the ear pinnae.*

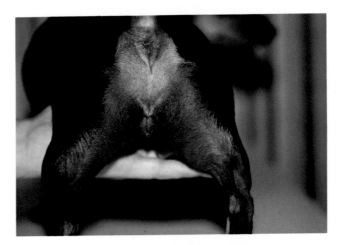

Figure 9-37 *Alopecia of caudal thighs with mild hyperpigmentation in 3-year-old female Dachshund.*

MISCELLANEOUS CANINE DERMATOSES

Acanthosis nigricans

Acral lick dermatitis (acral pruritic nodules, lick granulomas)

Anal sac disease

Bruises

Burns

Dalmation bronzing syndrome

Ear fissures

Eosinophilic granuloma (canine)

Flank sucking in Dobermans

Frostbite

Superficial necrolytic dermatitis (hepatic dermatopathy, "diabetic" dermatopathy)

Idiopathic lichenoid dermatitis

Mucinosis of the Chinese Shar Pei

Nasal solar dermatitis

Otitis externa

Paronychia (nail bed inflammation)

Perianal fistulas (perianal furunculosis)

Subcorneal pustular dermatosis (sterile neutrophilic pustular dermatosis)

Telogen defluxion (telogen effluvium)

Traction alopecia

Vitiligo-like disease (leukoderma)

Acanthosis Nigricans

CLINICAL SIGNS

1. Hyperpigmentation of the axillary areas
2. As the disease progresses the axillary areas usually become lichenified and seborrheic
3. In advanced cases the inguinal area, abdomen, ventral neck, and external ear canals may also be involved
4. Pruritus is variable; however, patients with secondary acanthosis are usually quite pruritic

DIAGNOSTIC AIDS

1. Clinical appearance is the most helpful diagnostic aid
2. Complete history
3. Skin biopsies for histopathologic examination are not diagnostic

The underlying etiology for primary acanthosis nigricans is unknown

UNDERLYING ETIOLOGIES (SECONDARY ACANTHOSIS NIGRICANS)

1. Axillary pruritus caused by allergic inhalant disease, food hypersensitivity, flea bite hypersensitivity, and contact dermatitis
2. Endocrine imbalances such as hypothyroidism and the various sex hormone imbalances
3. Seborrheic dermatoses, especially in Cocker Spaniels
4. Bacterial skin infection
5. Constant friction in the axillae caused by obesity or conformational abnormalities

COMMENTS

Primary acanthosis nigricans is an uncommon, hereditary disease and is seen mainly in Short-Haired Dachshunds. The age at onset is less than 1 year, and there is no sex predilection. Secondary acanthosis nigricans is a common manifestation of many canine skin diseases. Successful treatment of secondary acanthosis nigricans is based on treating the underlying etiology(ies).

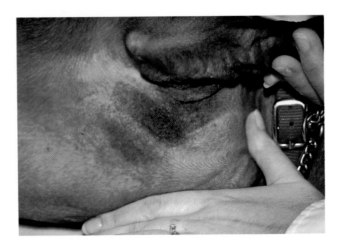

Figure 10-1   *Hyperpigmentation with some lichenification in right axillary area of 2-year-old Miniature Dachshund. Patient's disease started at 7 months of age.*

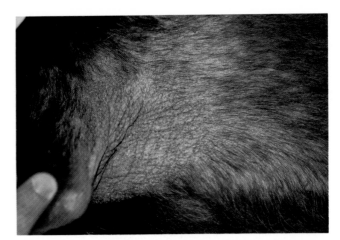

Figure 10-2   *Extensive hyperpigmentation with lichenification and some surrounding erythema in left axillary area of 5-year-old mixed-breed dog. Patient's acanthosis nigricans was secondary to pruritus caused by flea bite hypersensitivity.*

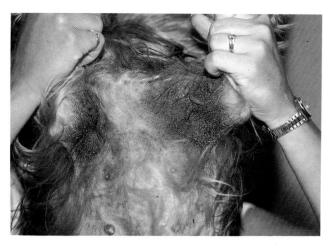

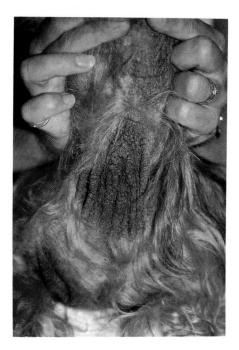

Figure 10-3   *Axillary area of 8-year-old Yorkshire Terrier. Hyperpigmentation and lichenification were secondary to pruritus caused by allergic inhalant disease.*

Figure 10-4   *Ventral neck of patient shown in Figure 10-3.*

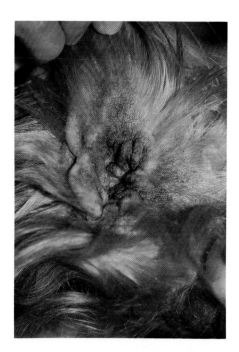

Figure 10-5   *Ear pinna and part of external ear canal of patient shown in Figures 10-3 and 10-4. Patient's otitis was secondary to inhalant allergies.*

Acral Lick Dermatitis (Acral Pruritic Nodules, Lick Granulomas)

CLINICAL SIGNS

1. The first sign is usually self-induced alopecia
2. This is followed by self-induced erosion of the epidermis, then ulceration
3. Chronic, self-induced trauma to the area leads to fibrosis and nodule formation

DIFFERENTIAL DIAGNOSIS

1. Pressure point granulomas
2. Deep bacterial infection
3. Mycotic granulomas
4. Dermatophyte infection
5. Neoplasia

UNDERLYING ETIOLOGIES

1. Allergic inhalant disease
2. Flea bite hypersensitivity
3. Foreign body
4. Hypothyroidism
5. Joint or bone pain
6. Neuritis
7. Psychological abnormalities; boredom

DIAGNOSTIC AIDS

1. Clinical appearance of the lesion
2. Skin biopsies for histopathologic examination may be quite helpful

COMMENTS

Acral pruritic dermatitis is a common presenting sign in many allergic patients. The most common sites are the anterior carpal, anterior metacarpal, and anterior metatarsal areas. The author has found the Golden Retriever, Labrador Retriever, Doberman Pinscher, Irish Setter, and German Shepherd Dog to be predisposed. Most patients are middle age bracket, and intact male dogs are slightly predisposed. Although it is frequently reported that "boredom" is the most common cause of acral pruritic dermatitis, the author believes that allergic inhalant disease is the most common underlying etiology.

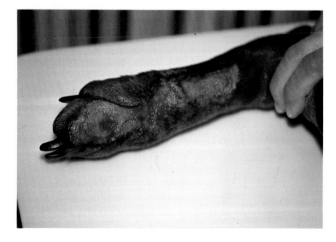

Figure 10-6 *Acral lick dermatitis on right rear leg of 6-year-old Doberman Pinscher. Patient's full-thickness epidermal defects were self-induced.*

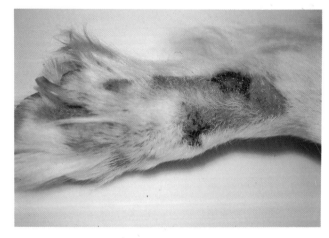

Figure 10-7 *Right rear leg of English Setter with allergic inhalant disease.*

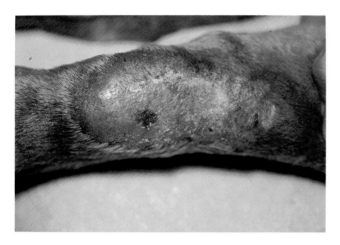

Figure 10-8   *Infected acral pruritic nodule on rear leg of 10-year-old Weimariner with hypothyroidism.*

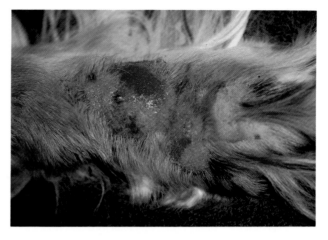

Figure 10-9   *Acral lick dermatitis on foreleg of mixed-breed dog. Underlying etiology for patient's self-induced trauma was allergic inhalant disease.*

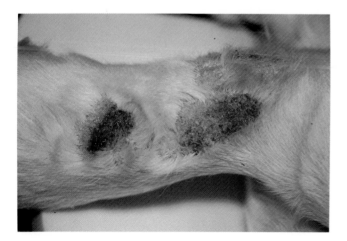

Figure 10-10   *Several acral pruritic "nodules" on rear leg of 5-year-old Saint Bernard. Patient's disease involved several limbs and most likely was secondary to hypothyroidism, flea bite hypersensitivity, and allergic inhalant disease.*

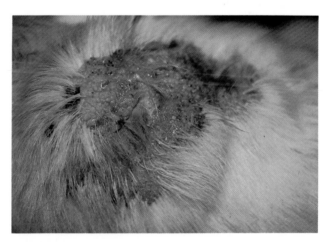

Figure 10-11   *Close-up of acral lick dermatitis on foreleg of patient shown in Figure 10-10.*

Anal Sac Disease

CLINICAL SIGNS

1. "Scooting" is the most common sign; however, many patients lick or bite the anal or tail base area
2. Areas of acute moist dermatitis may be found around the tail base due to the patient's attempts to alleviate the anal sac discomfort
3. The anal sac "area" may be erythematous, swollen, and/or abscessed

DIFFERENTIAL DIAGNOSIS

1. Patients with flea bite hypersensitivity, food hypersensitivity, and allergic inhalant disease often have rump, tail base, and anal area pruritus
2. Perianal fistulas may resemble anal sac abscessation and rupture
3. Perianal gland hyperplasia and/or tumors may resemble inflammation of the anal sacs
4. Anal sac tumors

DIAGNOSTIC AIDS

1. Clinical signs
2. Presence of an excessive amount of anal sac fluid or an anal sac secretion that is purulent or hemopurulent

COMMENTS

Anal sac inflammation, impaction, and abscessation should always be considered in patients showing signs of rear end pruritus. Smaller breeds of dogs may be predisposed. No age or sex predilection exists. Although cats do develop anal sac disease, it is much less common than in the dog. Predisposing factors include allergic, endocrine, and seborrheic skin disorders and changes in diet and fecal consistency.

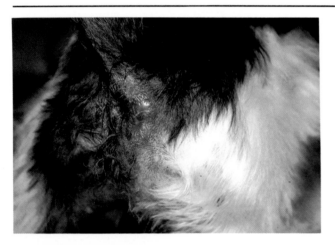

Figure 10-12   Abscess of right anal sac in young Lhasa Apso. Underlying etiology of patient's recurrent anal sacculitis and impaction was not known.

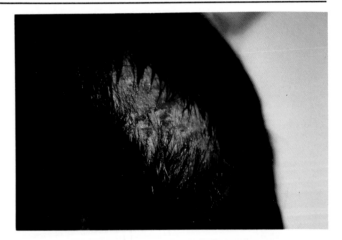

Figure 10-13   Four-year-old Labrador Retriever with area of acute moist dermatitis on hip, extending toward tail base. Patient's pruritus was caused by anal sac impaction.

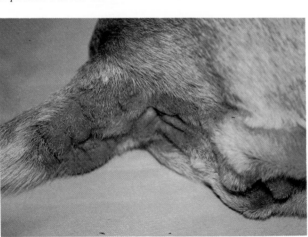

Figure 10-14   Erythema and lichenification of perianal area and ventral tail base of mixed Beagle. Patient's anal sacculitis and pruritus were caused by food hypersensitivity.

Bruises

CLINICAL SIGNS

1. Any area of the body may be involved, but owners are most likely to recognize a bruise on sparsely haired areas such as the abdomen and inguinal areas
2. Bruises are initially red in color, but over time they change to bluish purple or green
3. The size of a bruise depends upon the extent of the inciting trauma as well as the capability of the patient's clotting mechanisms and presence of diseases which may increase a patient's tendency to bruise

DIFFERENTIAL DIAGNOSIS

1. Hyperpigmentation associated with endocrine imbalances and self-trauma may resemble a bruise, but usually these conditions are easily differentiated by careful physical examination
2. Nevi and melanomas

DIAGNOSTIC AIDS

1. Careful clinical examination of the lesions
2. History is often helpful
3. Skin biopsies for histopathologic examination are rarely necessary and care should be taken when the lesion is extensive as the patient's clotting ability may be compromised

COMMENTS

Bruises are usually caused by blunt trauma, which may occur when the patient digs under or jumps over a fence, falls down stairs, or is hit by a car. Bruises are usually self-limiting; however, when the extent of the bruise appears to be excessive for the amount of sustained trauma, the patient's clotting ability should be assessed and possible underlying diseases which may increase a patient's tendency to bruise (such as hyperadrenocorticism) should be investigated.

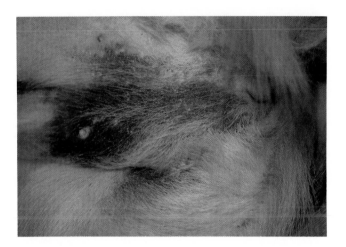

Figure 10-15 *Large bruise on abdomen of 13-year-old Shetland Sheepdog. This patient was injured when she fell down flight of stairs.*

Burns

CLINICAL SIGNS

1. The first sign of a burn is pain. This may be manifested by the patient licking the involved area. Initially, other signs are usually masked by the hair coat
2. Within 24 to 48 hours the involved skin becomes hard and dry
3. Bacterial infection and a purulent discharge often follow
4. Depending on the depth of the burn, areas of necrotic epidermis and dermis may slough, leaving a suppurating ulcer
5. Regrowth of hair and reepithelialization depend on the depth of the burn

DIFFERENTIAL DIAGNOSIS

1. Toxic epidermal necrolysis
2. Bullous pemphigoid
3. Pemphigus vulgaris

DIAGNOSTIC AIDS

1. Obviously if the burn was witnessed, history is extremely important
2. History of recent grooming (blow dryers and hot water) or surgery (heating pads) is suggestive
3. Clinical signs are very helpful but may be misleading

COMMENTS

The most common causes of burns in dogs are bath water that is too hot and blow dryers attached to the patient's cage. Other causes in dogs and cats include heating pads used during surgical procedures, hot car motors, caustic agents, and fires.

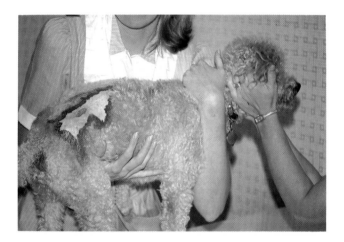

Figure 10-16   Healing burn on rump of 18-month-old Miniature Poodle. Trauma apparently occurred when patient was at groomers for bath and clip.

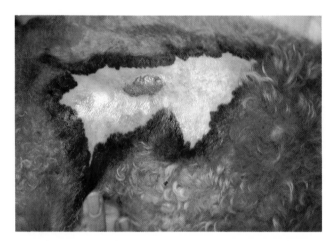

Figure 10-17   Closer view of burn shown in Figure 10-16. Central area is still in process of reepithelialization.

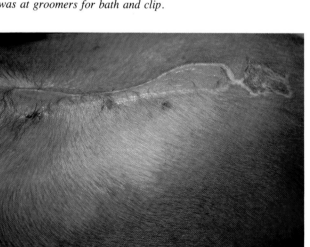

Figure 10-18   Longitudinal ulceration on abdomen of 7-year-old Miniature Dachshund. Lesion developed several days after patient underwent surgery for intervertebral disc disease. Burn was thought to have been caused by heating pad.

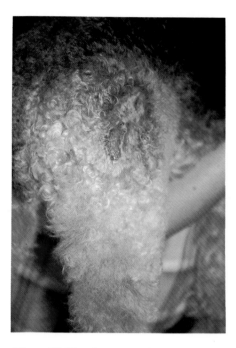

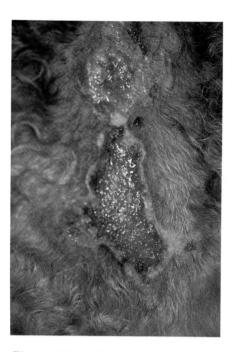

Figure 10-19   *Burn on right hip of Airedale Terrier. Injury was caused when patient was held against hot water pipe while being bathed.*

Figure 10-20   *Closer view of burn shown in Figure 10-19.*

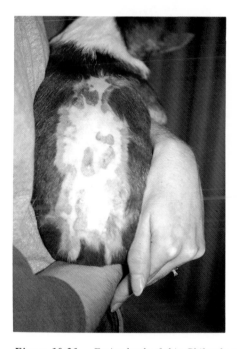

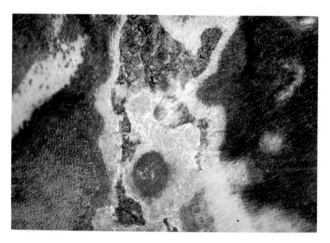

Figure 10-22   *Areas of erythema and necrosis on back of mixed-breed dog. Cause of this patient's extensive truncal burns was not determined.*

Figure 10-21   *Entire back of this Chihuahua is scarred after being burned by heating pad during ovariohysterectomy.*

Dalmatian Bronzing Syndrome

CLINICAL SIGNS

1. Dull, moth-eaten appearance to the haircoat
2. The entire trunk may be involved, but the most common area of involvement is the mid-back
3. The hair in involved areas is often a yellow to bronze color
4. Bacterial folliculitis of involved areas is common
5. Pruritus ranges from moderate to absent
6. In addition to cutaneous abnormalities, patients also have abnormal uric acid metabolism

DIFFERENTIAL DIAGNOSIS

1. Demodicosis
2. Food hypersensitivity
3. Allergic inhalant disease
4. Other causes of bacterial folliculitis
5. Other causes of urinary tract infections

DIAGNOSTIC AIDS

1. Breed of patient and location of lesions
2. Evaluation of patient's uric acid/purine metabolism
3. Response to a low-purine diet and medication

COMMENTS

Dalmatian bronzing syndrome is a rare disorder seen exclusively in Dalmatians. The disease is caused by an inherited metabolic defect in purine metabolism. High levels of uric acid are excreted directly into the urine; whereas in normal dogs the uric acid is converted and excreted as allantoin.

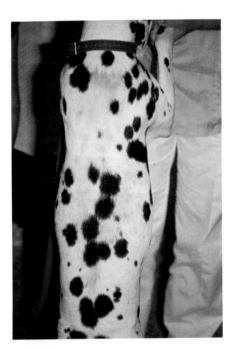

Figure 10-23 *Patchy partial alopecia with bacterial folliculitis on back of 20-month-old Dalmatian with Dalmatian bronzing syndrome.*

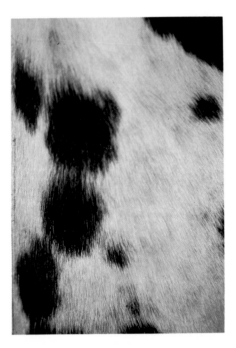

Figure 10-24 *Closer view of patient shown in Figure 10-23. Note light "bronze" color of coat.*

Ear Fissures

CLINICAL SIGNS

1. Ear fissures are tears in the ear pinnal edge, usually the distal margin, that result from self-trauma or underlying ear pinnal disease
2. Fissures may be very small defects (a few millimeters) or larger (2 to 3 cm) V-shaped defects
3. The trauma is induced either by head shaking or scratching with the hind leg(s)
4. Since the ear pinna is very vascular, marked hemorrhage is generally associated with these lesions

UNDERLYING ETIOLOGIES

1. Allergic otitis externa (caused by food, inhalant, and/or flea bite hypersensitivities)
2. *Otodectes cynotis* infestation
3. Fly strike ear pinnal damage
4. Sarcoptic mange
5. Cutaneous vasculitis
6. Ear margin seborrheic disease
7. Fight wounds

DIAGNOSTIC AIDS

1. Location and appearance of lesions
2. History of ear pinnal and periauricular pruritus or ear pinnal disease

COMMENTS

Ear (pinnal) fissures are seen in dogs suffering from head and ear pruritus, as well as in those with a history of ear pinnal disease. Flop-eared breeds, such as Dachshunds and Retrievers, are predisposed. Successful "treatment" (mainly in the form of prevention since severe ear fissures often require surgery) is based on detecting and treating the underlying etiology.

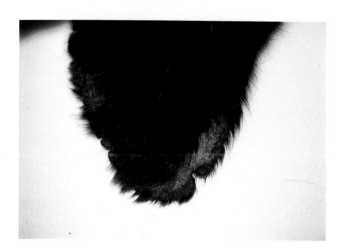

Figure 10-25 *Several small ear fissures on ear pinna of 6-year-old Labrador Retriever. Fissures were result of years of head shaking caused by otitis externa which was secondary to allergic inhalant disease.*

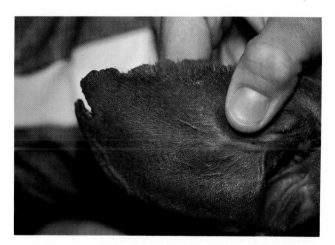

Figure 10-26 *Miniature Dachshund with ear pinnal fissures related to chronic ear margin sebborheic disease.*

Eosinophilic Granuloma (Canine)

CLINICAL SIGNS

1. The oral cavity and/or the skin may be involved
2. Oral cavity lesions are usually found on or under the tongue or on the soft palate
3. Lingual or sublingual lesions are proliferative masses that are frequently ulcerated
4. Palate lesions are circular, ulcerated plaques
5. Cutaneous lesions are often located on the abdomen, but any area of the body may be involved
6. Cutaneous lesions consist of papules, nodules, and plaques that may be ulcerated

DIFFERENTIAL DIAGNOSIS

1. Neoplasia
2. Other granulomatous diseases

DIAGNOSTIC AIDS

1. Clinical appearance and location of the lesions
2. Histopathologic examination of biopsy specimens reveals collagen degeneration, palisading granulomas, and an infiltrate consisting of eosinophils and histiocytes
3. Blood eosinophilia is not characteristic of this disease

COMMENTS

Canine eosinophilic granulomas are rare and are most frequently found in the oral cavity. Siberian Huskies are predisposed. Male dogs comprise about 70% of reported cases. Dogs under 4 years of age are predisposed. The etiology of this disease is not known. Cutaneous lesions may be a manifestation of various hypersensitivity diseases.

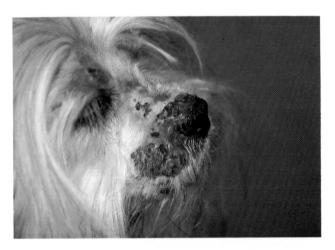

Figure 10-27 *Multiple eosinophilic granulomas on face and nose of young Lhasa Apso.*

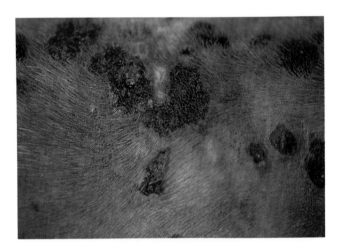

Figure 10-28 *Numerous eosinophilic granulomas on trunk of patient shown in Figure 10-27. Patient's disease responded totally to systemic corticosteroids.*

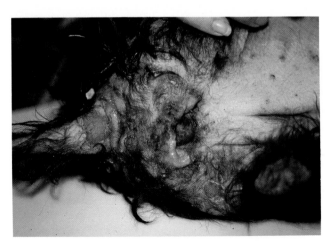

Figure 10-29 *Eroded eosinophilic granulomas involving perivulvar, perianal, and tail base areas of 4-year-old Poodle.*

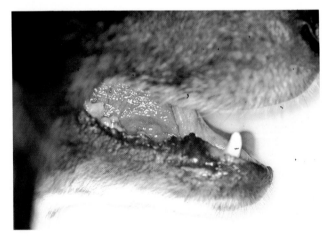

Figure 10-30 *Sublingual eosinophilic granuloma in Siberian Husky.*

Flank Sucking in Doberman Pinschers

CLINICAL SIGNS

1. Self-induced alopecia, often with erythema and/or hyperpigmentation
2. Lichenification of the involved skin may be seen in chronic cases
3. The flank is the area of involvement. In most cases the condition is unilateral; rarely it is bilateral

DIFFERENTIAL DIAGNOSIS

1. Allergic or hypersensitivity skin diseases including allergic inhalant disease, food hypersensitivity, flea bite hypersensitivity, and intestinal parasite hypersensitivity
2. Contact dermatitis

DIAGNOSTIC AIDS

1. Location of the "lesion"
2. Breed of dog involved

COMMENTS

Flank sucking is seen almost exclusively in the Doberman Pinscher. No age or sex predilection has been documented. The skin lesions seen in this condition are entirely self-induced. The underlying etiology appears to be a psychological aberration.

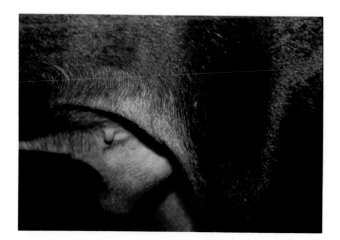

Figure 10-31   Young male Doberman Pinscher shows mild self-induced alopecia and lichenification of left flank. (Slide courtesy of Dr. William H. Miller, Ithaca, New York.)

Frostbite

CLINICAL SIGNS

1. Any area of the body may be involved, but the ear tips, tail tip, and scrotum are more commonly affected
2. Early signs are alopecia, erythema, and scaling of involved areas
3. Ulceration and necrosis with secondary bacterial infection develop

DIFFERENTIAL DIAGNOSIS

1. Various autoimmune or immune-mediated dermatoses, especially cold agglutinin disease and cutaneous vascultis
2. Fly strike dermatitis
3. Squamous cell carcinoma

DIAGNOSTIC AIDS

1. Distribution of lesions
2. Skin biopsies for histopathologic examination may be helpful
3. History of patient being exposed to temperatures below 30° C for prolonged periods of time

COMMENTS

Frostbite may be more common in weak or debilitated animals and in those patients not accustomed to exposure to extended periods of freezing temperatures. The condition is self-limiting when exposure to freezing temperatures is avoided. Permanent scarring often ensues; this is most evident on the ear pinnae, which may have a notched appearance.

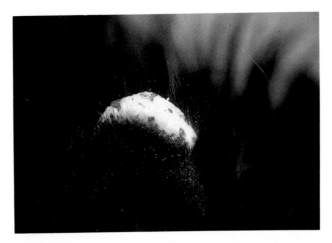

Figure 10-32 *Ear pinna of 16-year-old mixed German Shepherd Dog shows alopecia, erythema, and scaling. Patient's other ear pinna and tail tip were also involved.*

Superficial Necrolytic Dermatitis (Hepatic Dermatopathy, "Diabetic" Dermatopathy)

CLINICAL SIGNS

1. Erythematous, ulcerative crusting dermatitis
2. Areas of involvement include the face, mucocutaneous junctions, footpads, pressure points, and genitals
3. Hyperkeratosis of the footpads may be evident

DIFFERENTIAL DIAGNOSIS

1. Zinc dermatopathy
2. Pemphigus foliaceus
3. Pemphigus vulgaris
4. Systemic lupus erythematosus

DIAGNOSTIC AIDS

1. Complete physical examination
2. Chemistry profile, complete blood count, and urinalysis
3. Skin biopsies for histopathologic examination reveal superficial necrolytic dermatitis
4. Biopsies for direct immunofluorescence are negative
5. Exploratory surgery with biopsies of liver and careful search for pancreatic masses may be necessary

COMMENTS

Superficial necrolytic dermatitis was originally described as a diabetic dermatopathy, since the first documented cases had diabetes mellitus. It is now thought that the cutaneous abnormalities are associated with pancreatic tumors and/or hepatic disease. The disease has not been reported in the cat. Since this disease clinically resembles various autoimmune dermatoses, it is essential that a complete workup (including complete blood count, chemistry profile, and urinalysis) be performed on all patients suspected of having "autoimmune" skin disease.

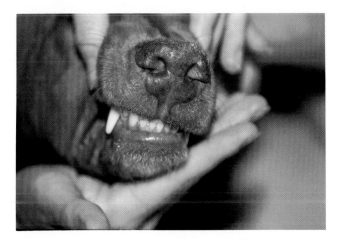

Figure 10-33   *Erythema with some erosions on muzzle and nose of 11-year-old mixed-breed dog with severe liver disease and diabetes mellitus.*

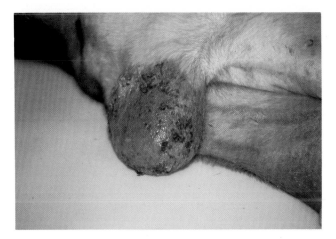

Figure 10-34   *Extensive scrotal ulceration on patient shown in Figure 10-33.*

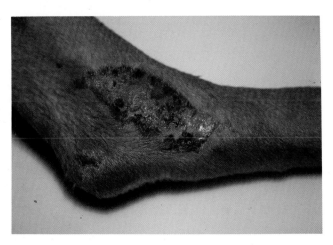

Figure 10-35   *Ulceration and crusting on lateral aspect of hock of patient shown in Figures 10-33 and 10-34.*

Idiopathic Lichenoid Dermatitis

CLINICAL SIGNS

1. Scaly and angular flat-topped papules
2. The papules typically develop into plaques
3. The lesions are often grouped or coalescing
4. Most lesions appear to be hyperkeratotic, and many are hyperpigmented
5. Lesions may be located anywhere on the body, including the face and ear pinnae
6. Lesions are asymptomatic (i.e., nonpruritic and nonpainful)

DIFFERENTIAL DIAGNOSIS

1. Bacterial dermatitis
2. Dermatophyte infection
3. Seborrheic dermatitis
4. Demodicosis

DIAGNOSTIC AIDS

1. Skin biopsies for histopathologic examination reveal some type of lichenoid interface dermatitis
2. Biopsies for direct immunofluorescence testing are negative
3. Lack of response to antibiotics, antifungals, and corticosteroids

COMMENTS

Idiopathic lichenoid dermatitis is an uncommon disorder in the dog. No age, breed, or sex predilection has been documented. The underlying etiology of the disease is not known; however, the clinical lesions appear to be the result of basal cell injury. (Many well-documented skin diseases are characterized histopathologically by lichenoid tissue reactions. These diseases include lupus erythematosus, forms of pemphigus, mycoses fungoides, and staphylococcal folliculitis.) Idiopathic lichenoid dermatitis spontaneously regresses in most cases.

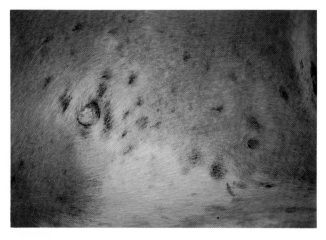

Figure 10-36 Numerous hyperpigmented, scaly plaques on lateral thorax of 5-year-old male Boxer with lichenoid dermatitis.

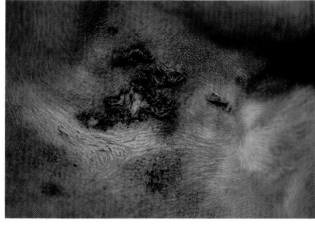

Figure 10-37 Coalescing, flat-topped papules in axillary area of patient shown in Figure 10-36.

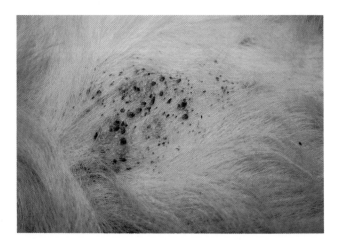

Figure 10-38 Axillary area of 8-year-old female mixed Collie shows flat-topped, hyperpigmented papules, and surrounding erythema.

Mucinosis of the Chinese Shar Pei

CLINICAL SIGNS

1. Affected dogs have puffy, swollen appearance especially on the head and extremities
2. The distal extremities may have a doughy feeling resembling pitting edema
3. Many patients actually have hundreds of cutaneous vesicles which contain a clear fluid
4. Patients are usually nonpruritic

DIAGNOSTIC AIDS

1. Breed of dog and clinical appearance of lesions
2. Skin biopsies for histopathologic examination are diagnostic

COMMENTS

Mucinosis is a common condition in the Chinese Shar Pei. (Some investigators feel that mucinosis is present in the skin of all Shar Pei's and that it is normal for the breed.) No sex predilection exists. Young animals are predisposed. The underlying etiology and the significance of this condition are not known.

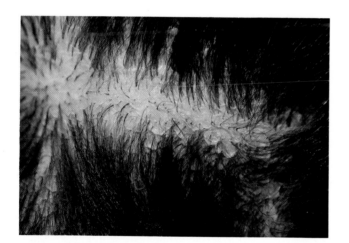

Figure 10-39 Axillary area of 10-month-old female Chinese Shar Pei shows numerous vesicles.

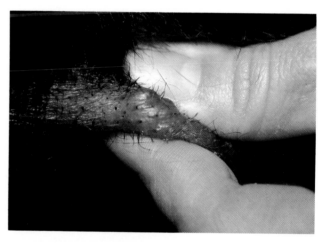

Figure 10-40 Vesicular lesions on rear leg of Shar Pei shown in Figure 10-39

Nasal Solar Dermatitis

CLINICAL SIGNS

1. Lesions occur on the planum nasale at the junction of haired and nonhaired skin in poorly pigmented patients
2. Alopecia, erythema, and scaling are present
3. The involved area may become crusted and/or ulcerated
4. Nasal erosion and/or squamous cell carcinoma may develop in chronic cases
5. Pruritus is mild to absent

DIFFERENTIAL DIAGNOSIS

1. Discoid lupus erythematosus
2. Systemic lupus erythematosus
3. Pemphigus foliaceous
4. Pemphigus erythematosus
5. Nasal pyoderma
6. Dermatomyositis
7. Dermatophyte infection
8. Demodicosis

DIAGNOSTIC AIDS

1. History of exposure to excessive ultraviolet radiation
2. Restriction of lesions to the nose
3. Biopsies for direct immunofluorescence testing are negative
4. Skin biopsies for histopathologic examination are helpful to rule out other differentials

COMMENTS

Nasal solar dermatitis is an uncommon cause of nasal dermatitis in the dog. Patients with poorly pigmented nasal skin living in sunny climates are predisposed. No age, breed, or sex predilections have been documented. Discoid lupus erythematosus and diseases of the pemphigus complex are frequently misdiagnosed as nasal solar dermatitis. This disease was formerly and inappropriately called "Collie nose". Most dermatoses on the nose of Collies and Shelties have an autoimmune basis.

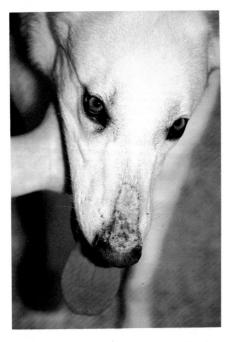

Figure 10-41 *Young German Shepherd Dog shows alopecia, erythema, and scaling of nose due to excessive exposure to sunlight.*

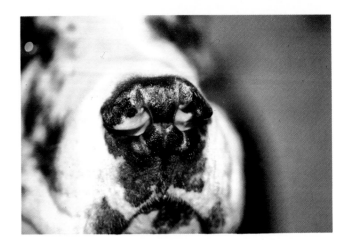

Figure 10-42 *Cracked, eroded nose of 3-year-old Great Dane caused by chronic actinic damage.*

Otitis Externa

CLINICAL SIGNS

1. Inflammation of the external ear canal and/or medial aspect of the ear pinna
2. Ulceration of the vertical and horizontal canals may be present in severe cases
3. The entire vertical canal may be swollen closed
4. An exudate is usually present that frequently has an offensive odor. The color of the exudate varies from whitish yellow to black. The consistency varies from slimy to caked and flaky
5. Pruritus and pain are manifested by head shaking as well as by rubbing and scratching the pinnae and periauricular areas

UNDERLYING ETIOLOGIES

1. Allergic inhalant disease (atopy)
2. Food hypersensitivity
3. Flea bite hypersensitivity
4. *Otodectes cynotis* infestation-ear mites
5. Demodectic mites
6. Structural "defects" such as heavy, floppy ear pinnae
7. Irritating chemicals/drugs or water placed in the external ear canal
8. Foreign bodies such as foxtails
9. Autoimmune or immune-mediated dermatoses may have ear pinnal and/or external ear canal involvement
10. Neoplastic disease
11. Primary bacterial or fungal infection

DIAGNOSTIC AIDS

1. Complete otoscopic examination of the horizontal and vertical canals and tympanum
2. Cytologic examination of ear exudate
3. Culture and sensitivity of exudate
4. Biopsy of pinna and/or external canal may be helpful in some cases

COMMENTS

Otitis externa is a common component of many canine dermatologic disorders. It is much less common in the cat. Age, breed, and sex predilections vary according to the underlying etiology. Primary bacterial or fungal otitis externa is quite rare. Successful treatment depends upon detection and treatment of the underlying etiology.

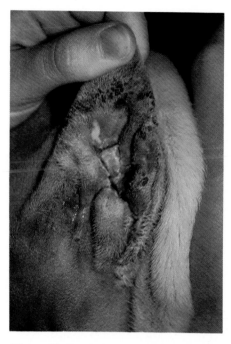

Figure 10-43   *Inflamed and crusted ear pinna of 2-year-old Chinese Shar Pei with food hypersensitivity and allergic inhalant disease. Note purulent exudate. Opening of external ear canal is swollen closed.*

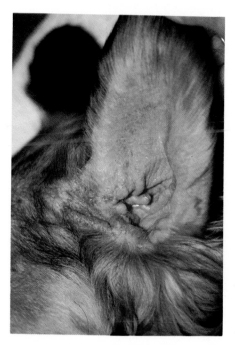

Figure 10-44   *Marked inflammation with some hyperpigmentation of medial aspect of ear pinna and periauricular area of mixed-breed dog with allergic inhalant disease (atopy).*

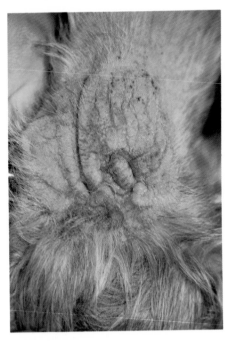

Figure 10-45 *Crusting, erythema, hyperpigmentation, and lichenification of ear pinna of Lhasa Apso with food hypersensitivity.*

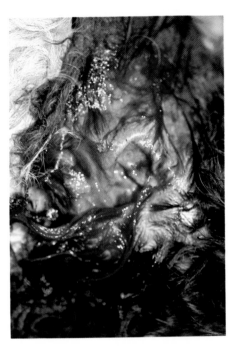

Figure 10-46 *Ulceration and mucoid exudate of ear pinna of 13-year-old mixed-breed dog with cutaneous lymphoma. This inflammatory process involved entire external ear canal.*

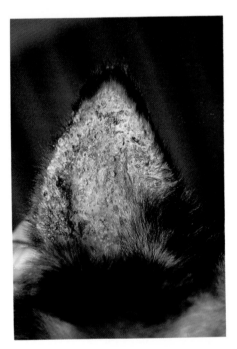

Figure 10-47 *Scaling and crusting on ear pinna of young male Akita with pemphigus foliaceus. Several pustules are seen in center of pinna.*

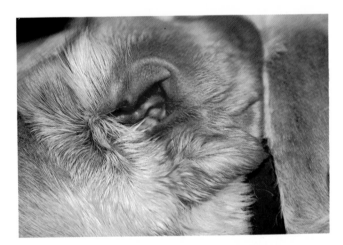

Figure 10-48 *Severe erythema of ear pinna, extending down vertical ear canal, of 4-year-old yellow Labrador Retriever with adverse drug reaction to sulfa/trimethoprim antibiotic.*

Paronychia (Nail Bed Inflammation)

CLINICAL SIGNS

1. Erythema, swelling, and in some cases ulceration of the tissue surrounding the nail(s)
2. A purulent discharge may be present
3. In most cases paronychia results in some type of deformity of the nail itself
4. The nail may be shed from the nail bed
5. Pain is usually present and is manifested by licking the foot (feet) and/or limping

UNDERLYING ETIOLOGIES

1. Bacterial infection
2. Fungal infection
3. Demodicosis
4. Autoimmune or immune-mediated diseases
5. Foreign body
6. Neoplasia

DIAGNOSTIC AIDS

1. Skin scrapings for demodectic mites
2. Culture and sensitivity testing of the exudate
3. Fungal culture of the nail itself
4. Biopsy of the nail bed for histopathologic examination and immunofluorescence testing

COMMENTS

Paronychia is a component of many canine and feline dermatologic disorders. One, several, or all of the nail beds may be involved. As with most skin diseases, successful treatment depends on identifying and treating the underlying etiology.

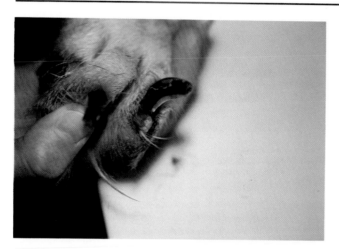

Figure 10-49   *Nail lifting from nail bed on forefoot of 6-year-old German Shepherd Dog with pemphigus vulgaris.*

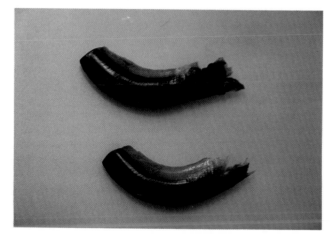

Figure 10-50   *Two nails removed from patient shown in Figure 10-49.*

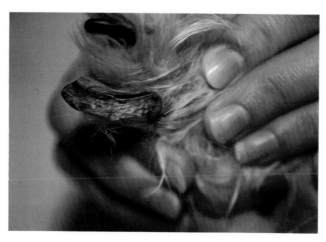

Figure 10-51   *Severely distorted nail with inflamed nail bed on forefoot of 12-year-old mixed-breed dog. Histopathology of mass from involved toe revealed malignant melanoma.*

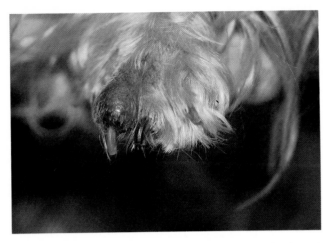

Figure 10-52 *Marked inflammation of third toe on forefoot of 15-year-old Yorkshire Terrier. Underlying etiologies for patient's paronychia were demodicosis and bacterial infection.*

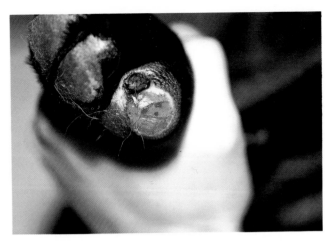

Figure 10-53 *Ulcerated granulomatous lesion involving nail bed of Labrador Retriever. Etiology was thought to be a foreign body.*

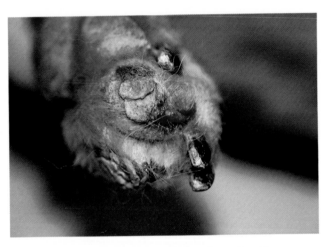

Figure 10-54 *Hyperkeratotic, peeling footpads with paronychia on forefoot of 7-year-old mixed-breed dog with pemphigus vulgaris.*

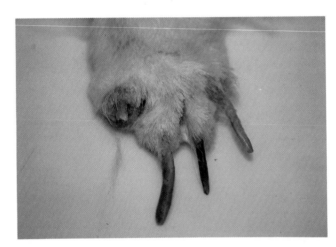

Figure 10-55 *Deformed nails on forefoot of 10-year-old Shetland Sheepdog with* Trichophyton mentagrophytes *infection.*

Perianal Fistulas (Perianal Furunculosis)

CLINICAL SIGNS

1. Ulceration of the perianal area with fistulous tracts
2. Necrosis of the epidermis is usually present
3. Granulation tissue formation and fibrosis are commonly seen
4. Lesions are quite painful
5. Pruritus is usually mild

DIFFERENTIAL DIAGNOSIS

1. Autoimmune disease
2. Anal sac rupture
3. Neoplasia
4. Trauma

DIAGNOSTIC AIDS

1. Classic clinical appearance
2. Skin biopsies for histopathologic examination are usually diagnostic but may not be necessary

COMMENTS

Perianal fistulas are found almost exclusively in German Shepherd Dogs and their crosses. However, the disease has been reported in other breeds including Great Danes, Irish Setters, English Springer Spaniels, and English Setters. Older dogs appear to be predisposed. Intact male dogs may be predisposed. The etiology of this disease is not clear; however, poor ventilation of the perianal area in breeds with broad tails seems to be a major factor.

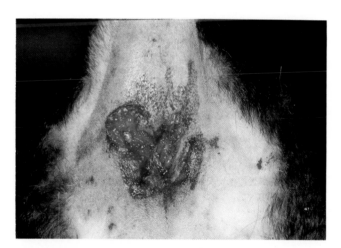

Figure 10-56   *Ulceration of perianal area of 4-year-old female spayed German Shepherd Dog with perianal fistulas. (Slide courtesy of Dr. David Saylor, Gaithersburg, Maryland.)*

Subcorneal Pustular Dermatosis (Sterile Neutrophilic Pustular Dermatosis)

CLINICAL SIGNS

1. Multiple pustules, yellow to yellowish-green in color, are the earliest clinical signs
2. Pustules range in size from approximately 2 mm to 1.5 cm in diameter and are nonfollicular
3. Older lesions are manifested by circular areas of alopecia, scaling, and crusting
4. Any area of the body may be involved, but the trunk, especially the axillary and inguinal areas, may be predisposed
5. Pruritus is variable

DIFFERENTIAL DIAGNOSIS

1. Pemphigus foliaceus or pemphigus vegetans
2. Bacterial folliculitis
3. Allergic diseases that have secondary bacterial or pustular lesions, these include allergic inhalant disease, food hypersensitivity, and flea bite hypersensitivity
4. Demodicosis
5. Dermatophyte infection

DIAGNOSTIC AIDS

1. Skin biopsies for histopathologic examination reveals subcorneal (intraepidermal) pustules containing neutrophils and occasional acantholytic keratinocytes
2. Biopsies for direct immunofluorescence testing is negative
3. Bacterial cultures of intact pustules are negative
4. Response to dapsone (Avlosulfon)

COMMENTS

Subcorneal pustular dermatosis is a rare, superficial pustular disease of dogs. No age, breed, or sex predilection has been documented. No underlying etiology has been detected. This disease is not responsive to systemic corticosteroids or antibiotics. It is the author's belief that many cases that are labeled subcutaneous pustular dermatoses are actually unusual or poorly responsive forms of pemphigus foliaceus.

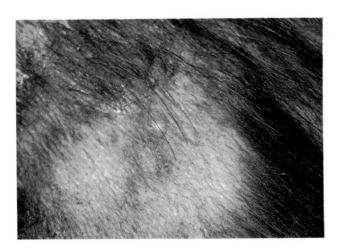

Figure 10-57   *Pustules on lateral thoracic area of middle-aged mixed German Shepherd Dog. Cultures of lesions were negative for bacteria.*

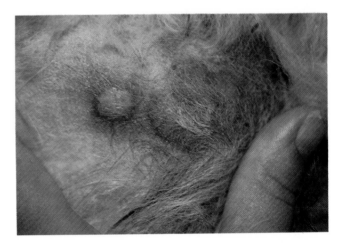

Figure 10-58   *Pustules on abdomen of 11-year-old Maltese. Cultures for bacteria were negative and histopathology revealed subcorneal pustules with neutrophils.*

Telogen Defluxion (Telogen Effluvium)

CLINICAL SIGNS

1. Acute, dramatic "shedding" of hairs mainly on the trunk
2. The abnormal shed usually results in areas of patchy, total or near-total alopecia
3. Remaining hairs are usually easily epilated
4. The skin in involved areas appears normal
5. Patients are nonpruritic

DIFFERENTIAL DIAGNOSIS

1. Endocrine imbalances
2. Normal shedding
3. Excessive shedding

UNDERLYING ETIOLOGIES

1. Anesthesia/surgery
2. Vaccinations
3. Drugs
4. Shock
5. Severe illness
6. Pregnancy and/or lactation

DIAGNOSTIC AIDS

1. Complete history and physical examination
2. Microscopic examination of hairs plucked from involved areas is often diagnostic

COMMENTS

Telogen defluxion is an uncommon cause of hair loss in the dog. The hair loss usually occurs within a very short period of time (less than 72 hours) and is often quite dramatic. No age or breed predilections have been documented. Pregnant or nursing females appear to be predisposed. Normal hair regrowth usually occurs within 1 to 3 months.

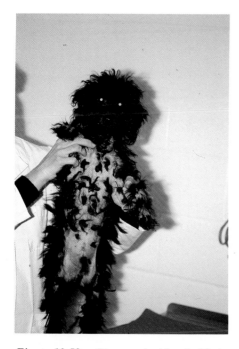

Figure 10-59   *Five-month-old male Miniature Poodle shows patchy, truncal alopecia which occurred within 7 days after third distemper/hepatitis/leptospirosis vaccination.*

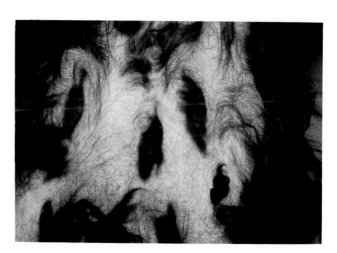

Figure 10-60   *Closer view of patient shown in Figure 10-59.*

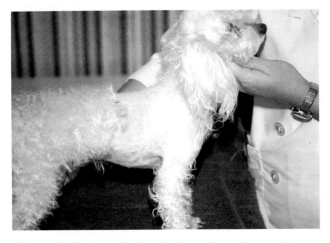

Figure 10-61   *Partial alopecia of shoulders, chest, and thorax in 11-month-old female Poodle following ovariohysterectomy.*

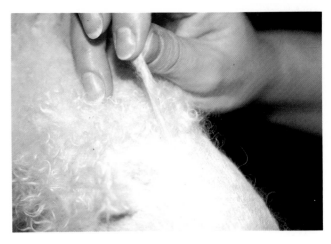

Figure 10-62   *Photo depicting easy epilation of truncal hair on patient shown in Figure 10-61.*

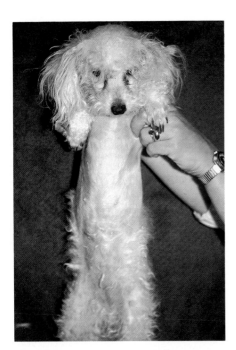

Figure 10-63   *Alopecic ventrum of patient shown in Figures 10-61 and 10-62. Patient regrew normal haircoat within 3 months after initiation of telogen effluvium.*

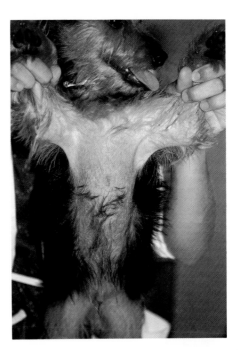

Figure 10-64   *Near-total alopecia of axillae and chest of young Silky Terrier possibly caused by deworming medication. (Area of erythema is sight of skin scraping.)*

Traction Alopecia

CLINICAL SIGNS

1. Alopecia may occur in areas where rubber bands or barretts are placed in the hair for ornamental purposes. Usually these devices were applied too tightly or actually pinched the skin in the band or barrett
2. The most common areas of involvement are the top of the head and the base of the ears
3. The alopecia is often permanent
4. Skin in involved areas may be hyperpigmented
5. Patients may be pruritic initially when the ornamental device is causing discomfort; however, once the alopecia occurs patients are not pruritic

DIFFERENTIAL DIAGNOSIS

1. Dermatophyte infection
2. Demodicosis
3. Other trauma

DIAGNOSTIC AIDS

1. Breed of patient and knowlege of past grooming techniques
2. Location and appearance of lesion
3. Skin biopsies for histopathologic examination may show follicular atrophy

COMMENTS

Traction alopecia is an uncommon cause of hair loss in the dog. It is most frequently seen at the base of the ears in Poodles and other breeds that have ornamental devices such as bows and barretts attached to the hair (and possibly skin) at the base of the ears. It is also seen on the top knot in Yorkshire Terriers, Silky Terriers, Lhasa Apsos and Shih Tzus who have bows and/or barretts attached to the hairs in the top of the head. The alopecia is usually permanent.

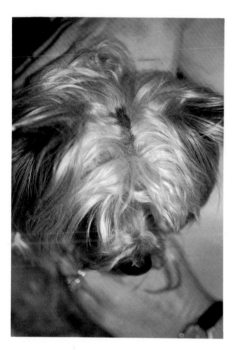

Figure 10-65 Alopecia with hyperpigmentation on the head of Silky Terrier. Patient's permanent alpecia was caused by repeated application of a rubber band and barrett that was used to keep hair out of eyes.

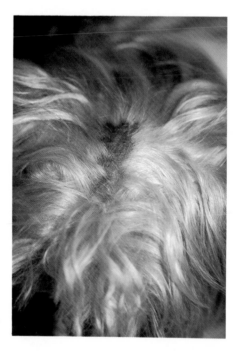

Figure 10-66 Closer view of alopecic area shown in Figure 10-65

Vitiligo-like Disease (Leukoderma)

CLINICAL SIGNS

1. Patchy depigmentation and/or hypopigmentation
2. This condition is most frequently seen on the nose, lips, and periocular areas; however, any area of the body may be involved
3. Pruritus, pain, and signs of systemic disease are absent

DIFFERENTIAL DIAGNOSIS

1. Discoid lupus erythematosus
2. Systemic lupus erythematosus
3. Vogt-Koyanagi-Harada-like syndrome
4. Lymphosarcoma (mycoses fungoides)
5. Contact dermatitis (especially due to plastic food dishes), may result in pigment loss

DIAGNOSTIC AIDS

1. Skin biopsies for histopathologic examination are helpful but may not be necessary
2. Careful examination reveals that the involved skin or mucous membrane is normal (no scales, crusts, erosions, or ulcerations) other than the pigment loss

COMMENTS

Vitiligo-like disease is a relatively common abnormality in the dog. No age, breed, or sex predilection exists. No underlying etiology has been detected. In some cases the involved areas spontaneously repigment.

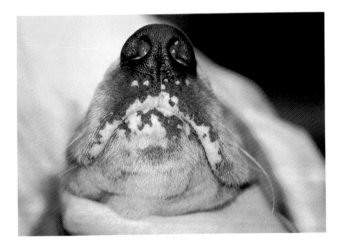

Figure 10-67 Patchy hypopigmentation of lips of 2-year-old Golden Retriever. Patient had normal black pigment in these areas until 3 months prior to presentation.

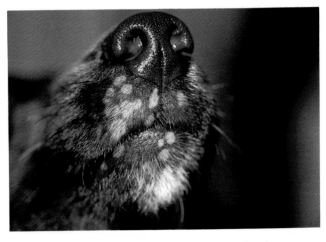

Figure 10-68 Hypopigmented patches on muzzle of 18-month-old male Shetland Sheepdog.

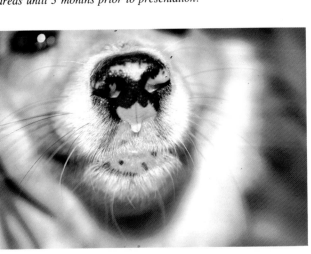

Figure 10-69 Patchy hypopigmentation of nose and lips of middle-aged mixed-breed female dog.

MISCELLANEOUS FELINE DERMATOSES

Eosinophilic plaque (eosinophilic granuloma, feline lick granuloma)

Eosinophilic ulcer (rodent ulcer, indolent ulcer)

Linear granuloma

Feline "endocrine" alopecia

Head and neck excoriations (head and neck pruritus)

Hyperesthesia syndrome

Miliary dermatitis

Neurodermatitis (feline psychogenic alopecia, feline psychogenic dermatitis)

Plasma cell pododermatitis

Preauricular alopecia

Self-induced alopecia

Eosinophilic Plaque (Eosinophilic Granuloma, Feline Lick Granuloma)

CLINICAL SIGNS

1. Raised, ulcerated plaques or plaquelike lesions that often coalesce
2. Lesions are most frequently located on the abdomen and medial thighs
3. Lesions are quite pruritic and are actually self-induced and self-perpetuated

DIFFERENTIAL DIAGNOSIS

1. Neoplasia
2. Infectious or foreign body granulomas
3. Deep fungal infections

UNDERLYING ETIOLOGIES

1. Allergic inhalant disease (atopy)
2. Food hypersensitivity
3. Flea bite hypersensitivity
4. Contact hypersensitivity

DIAGNOSTIC AIDS

1. History, appearance, and location of lesion(s)
2. Skin biopsies for histopathologic examination show hyperplastic, superficial, and deep perivascular dermatitis with eosinophilia or diffuse eosinophilic dermatitis
3. A complete blood count usually reveals eosinophilia

COMMENTS

Eosinophilic plaques are commonly seen in cats. These lesions are self-induced and in most cases are caused by an underlying allergic or hypersensitivity disease. Some cases are "idiopathic" and may be a manifestation of a psychological abnormality. No age, breed, or sex predilection has been documented.

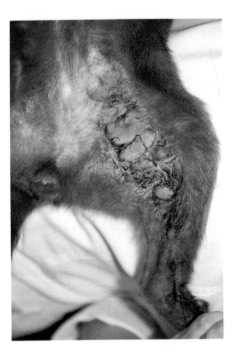

Figure 11-1   *Medial aspect of left rear leg of 3-year-old Domestic Short-Haired cat shows several glistening, coalescing eosinophilic plaques.*

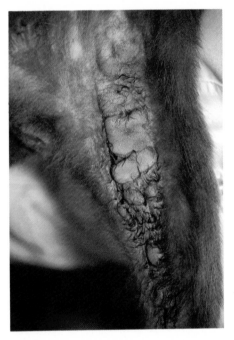

Figure 11-2   *Caudal aspect of right rear leg of patient shown in Figure 11-1. Underlying etiology for patient's numerous eosinophilic plaques was allergic inhalant disease.*

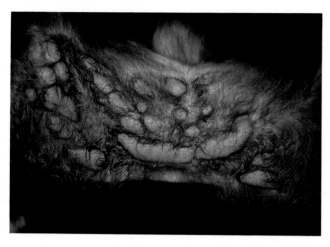

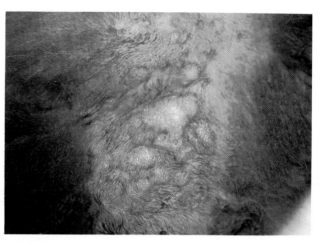

Figure 11-3 Abdomen of 5-year-old Domestic Short-Haired cat with several eosinophilic plaques. This patient's disease was caused by flea bite hypersensitivity.

Figure 11-4 Nine-year-old long-haired cat with eosinophilic plaque lesions on medial aspect of left rear leg. Patient was suffering from allergic inhalant disease.

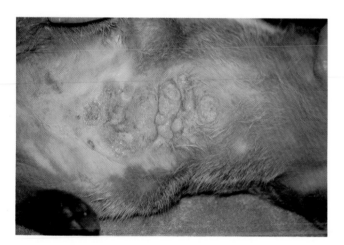

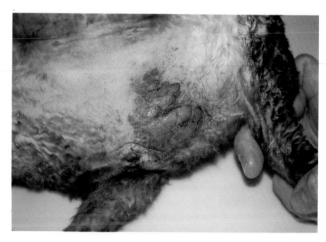

Figure 11-5 Abdomen of 8-year-old Abyssinian cat shows numerous, large, coalescing eosinophilic plaques.

Figure 11-6 Large eosinophilic plaque in inguinal area of 3-year-old Rex cat. Food hypersensitivity was determined to be cause of this patient's disease.

Eosinophilic Ulcer (Rodent Ulcer, Indolent Ulcer)

CLINICAL SIGNS

1. The most common clinical sign is varying degrees of ulceration of the upper lip
2. The lower lip, hard palate, and soft palate may also be involved
3. Chronic lip lesions may progress to squamous cell carcinoma
4. Lesions may be painful, and in severe cases the patient may be anorectic

DIFFERENTIAL DIAGNOSIS

1. Neoplasia
2. Autoimmune or immune-mediated skin disease

DIAGNOSTIC AIDS

1. Location and appearance of the lesion(s)
2. Skin biopsies for histopathologic examination show hyperplastic, perivascular dermatitis with neutrophils, plasma cells, and mononuclear cells
3. Blood and tissue eosinophilia are rarely found
4. Most patients are negative for feline leukemia virus

COMMENTS

Eosinophilic ulcers are commonly seen in the cat. No age, breed, or sex predilection has been documented. The underlying etiology is not known. However, the author believes that in some cases, especially those with both eosinophilic ulcers and eosinophilic granulomas, an underlying allergic disease is the precipitating factor. It has been reported that eosinophilic ulcers are often associated with feline leukemia virus; however, the author has found most patients to be FeLv negative.

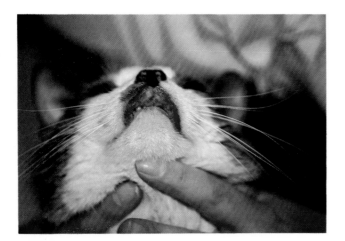

Figure 11-7 *Extensive ulceration of upper lip of male Domestic Short-Haired cat.*

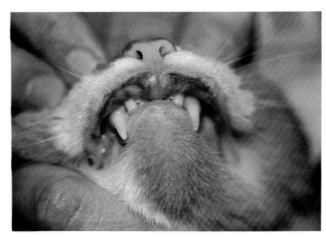

Figure 11-8 *Eosinophilic ulcer on upper lip of 4-year-old mixed-breed cat. This patient also had eosinophilic plaques on abdomen.*

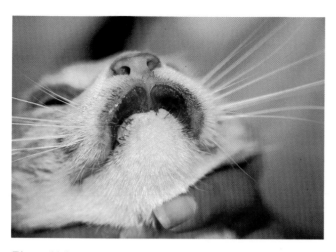

Figure 11-9   *Five-year-old long-haired cat with swollen, hemorrhagic, and very painful eosinophilic ulcer.*

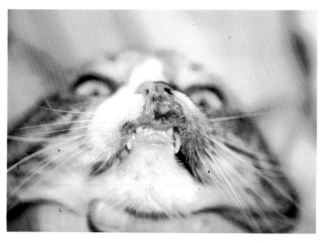

Figure 11-10   *Squamous cell carcinoma of upper lip of 13-year-old cat. Patient had 6-year history of "rodent ulcers."*

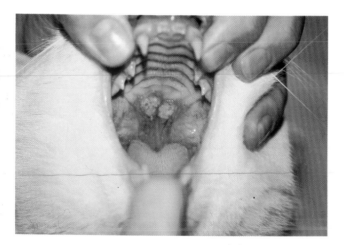

Figure 11-11   *Eosinophilic ulcers on soft palate of young mixed-breed cat.*

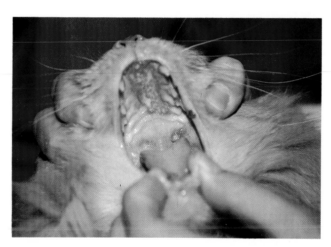

Figure 11-12   *Advanced eosinophilic ulcer on hard palate of 10-year-old cat. A smaller ulcer is seen on soft palate.*

Linear Granuloma

CLINICAL SIGNS

1. Raised, chordlike, yellow to pink linear plaques
2. Lesions are usually on the caudal aspects of the rear legs
3. Occasionally the axillary areas, forelegs, chin, and oral cavity are involved
4. Lesions are generally asymptomatic; however, some patients show varying degrees of pruritus

DIFFERENTIAL DIAGNOSIS

1. Neoplasia
2. Foreign body or infectious granulomas

DIAGNOSTIC AIDS

1. Location and appearance of the lesion(s)
2. Skin biopsies for histopathologic examination show nodular-to-diffuse dermatitis caused by granulomatous inflammation with collagen degeneration. Tissue eosinophilia may be present
3. Blood eosinophilia may be seen in patients with oral lesions

COMMENTS

Linear granulomas are the least common form of the eosinophilic granuloma complex. No breed or sex predilection exists. Young cats may be predisposed. An underlying etiology has not been determined.

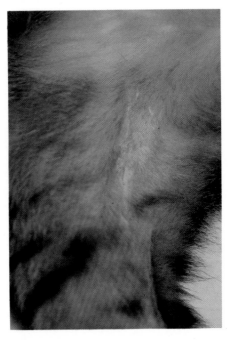

Figure 11-13 *Linear granuloma on caudomedial aspect of right rear leg of 2-year-old Calico cat.*

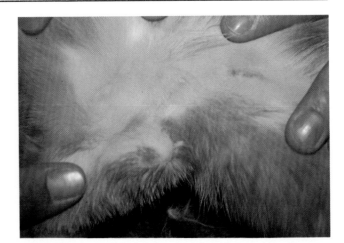

Figure 11-14 *Several linear granulomas in axillary area of young male Domestic Short-Haired cat. Owner reported that cat occasionally licked area. (Hair in involved area was shaved.)*

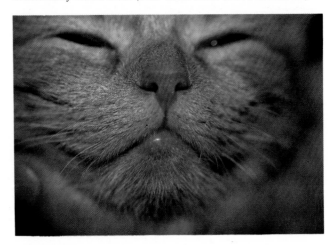

Figure 11-15 *Linear granuloma on lower lip of patient shown in Figure 11-14.*

Feline "Endocrine" Alopecia

CLINICAL SIGNS

1. Bilaterally symmetric hair loss which often begins in the perineal area
2. Other areas of involvement include the abdomen, caudomedial thighs, lateral thorax, and forelimbs
3. The hair loss is not a complete alopecia of involved areas, but rather a diffuse thinning
4. Patients are not pruritic

DIFFERENTIAL DIAGNOSIS

1. Allergic inhalanat disease
2. Food hypersensitivity
3. Flea bite hypersensitivity
4. Neurodermatitis
5. Hyperthyroidism

DIAGNOSTIC AIDS

1. Rule out other differentials via appropriate diagnostic tests
2. Microscopic examination of hairs plucked from involved areas. (If alopecia is self-induced and therefore not feline endocrine alopecia, the hair bulbs will be normal and ends of the hair shafts will be frayed
3. Skin biopsies for histopathologic examination may help to rule out other differentials

COMMENTS

Feline endocrine alopecia is a rare cause of hair loss in the cat. Common allergic diseases are often misdiagnosed as feline endocrine alopecia because the owners do not observe the patient licking the hair out. It is essential to take a careful history and microscopically examine hairs to determine if the hair loss is self-induced. REMEMBER, the hair loss in feline endocrine alopecia patients is *not* self-induced. The etiology of this disease is unknown. No age or breed predilection exists. Neutered males may be predisposed.

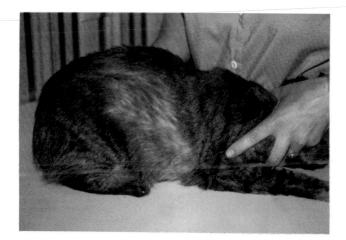

Figure 11-16 *Three-year-old neutered male cat with non-self-induced hair loss on lateral thorax. Alopecic pattern was bilaterally symmetric.*

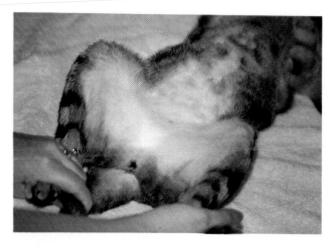

Figure 11-17 *Extensive alopecia on abdomen and medial thighs of seven-year-old male neutered cat.*

Head and Neck Excoriations (Head and Neck Pruritus)

CLINICAL SIGNS

1. Varying degrees of self-induced alopecia, papules, and excoriations involving the head and/or neck
2. The degree of pruritus varies according to the underlying etiology
3. The extent of self-induced damage often varies depending upon the presence or absence of claws and the personality of the patient. (Hyperactive, fidgity cats usually inflict more damage than calm, placid ones.)

UNDERLYING ETIOLOGIES

1. *Otodectes cynotes* (ear mites)
2. Notoedric mange
3. Allergic inhalant disease
4. Food hypersensitivity
5. Flea bite hypersensitivity
6. *Cheyletiella* infestation
7. Dermatophyte infection
8. Flea collar dermatitis

DIAGNOSTIC AIDS

1. Appearance and location of the lesions
2. Skin scrapings are necessary in all cases
3. Fungal culture for dermatophyte infection
4. Intradermal skin testing for allergic inhalant disease
5. Allergy test diet consisting of lamb and bottled water for 4 weeks

COMMENTS

Head and neck excoriations are frequently seen in feline patients with pruritic skin disease. No age, breed, or sex predilection exists. As with most skin diseases, successful treatment depends on detecting and treating the underlying cause(s).

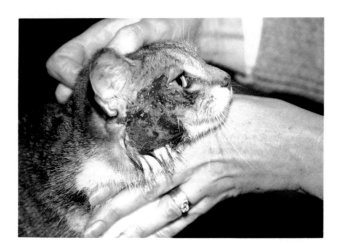

Figure 11-18 *Extensive excoriation on face of 5-year-old Domestic Short-Haired cat with food hypersensitivity.*

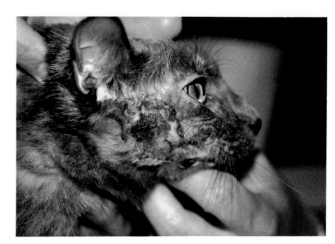

Figure 11-19 *Excoriated cheek of 6-year-old female cat with allergic inhalant disease. Patient also had eosinophilic plaques on abdomen.*

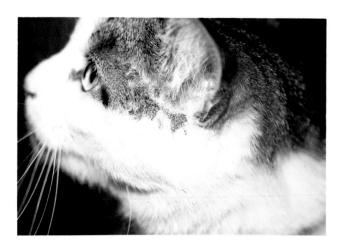

Figure 11-20   *Domestic Short-Haired cat with preauricular excoriations. Patient's pruritus was caused by flea bite hypersensitivity.*

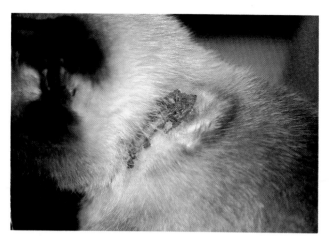

Figure 11-21   *Young male Siamese cat with excoriated areas on neck. Underlying cause of patient's pruritus was allergic inhalant disease.*

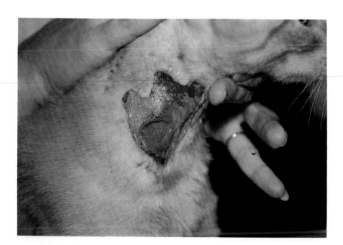

Figure 11-22   *Two-year-old cat with severely excoriated neck has exposed muscle tissue caused by flea bite hypersensitivity.*

Hyperesthesia Syndrome

CLINICAL SIGNS

1. Aberrant behavior includes the following: licking and biting of body parts, especially the chest and forelegs; tail chasing; skin rippling and muscle spasms; sensitivity over the lumbar area; wild running and jumping; growling and other vocalizations
2. Stimuli, especially petting over the lumbar area, will often induce the signs in a patient

DIFFERENTIAL DIAGNOSIS

1. Estrus
2. Rabies
3. Neuritis/arthritis
4. Lead toxicity
5. Anal gland impaction
6. Psychomotor epilepsy

DIAGNOSTIC AIDS

1. Characteristic, unusual behavior
2. All laboratory tests, including skin biopsies and electroencephalograms are normal

COMMENTS

Feline hyperesthesia is relatively common. There is no age, breed, or sex predilection. The underlying etiologies have not been determined. Cutaneous abnormalities often result when the aberrant behavior causes excessive licking or biting of a particular area on the animal.

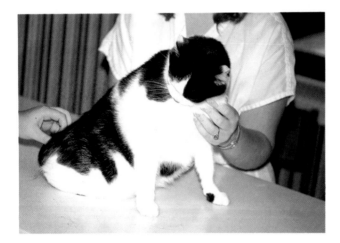

Figure 11-23   *Nine-year-old male Domestic Short-Haired cat. Rubbing this patient's lumbar area caused immediate, compulsive licking and biting of shoulder and chest areas.*

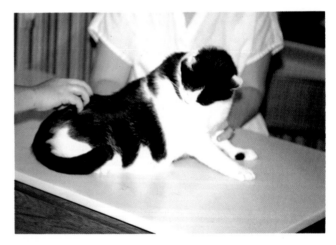

Figure 11-24   *Another photograph of hyperesthetic patient shown in Figure 11-23.*

Miliary Dermatitis

CLINICAL SIGNS

1. Pruritic papules on the trunk, especially the mid-back
2. Varying degrees of self-induced alopecia may be present
3. The papules may be excoriated and covered by crusts
4. Pruritus may vary from mild to severe

UNDERLYING ETIOLOGIES

1. Flea bite hypersensitivity
2. Food hypersensitivity
3. Allergic inhalant disease
4. Intestinal parasitism
5. *Cheyletiella* infestation
6. Dermatophyte infection
7. Pediculosis
8. Chiggers
9. Bacterial folliculitis
10. Drug eruption
11. Idiopathic

DIAGNOSTIC AIDS

1. Appearance of lesions
2. Close examination to check for fleas, flea excreta, lice, and tapeworm segments
3. Skin scrapings are essential
4. Dermatophyte culture
5. Skin biopsies for histopathologic examination may be helpful
6. Allergy test diet
7. Intradermal skin testing for allergic inhalant disease

COMMENTS

Miliary dermatitis is a very common manifestation of many feline dermatologic disorders. Flea bite hypersensitivity is considered to be the major cause of miliary dermatitis. No age, breed, or sex predilection exists. The underlying etiology can be detected in most patients with miliary dermatitis by careful history taking, physical examination, and selected diagnostic procedures. Again, successful treatment must be directed at the underlying etiology.

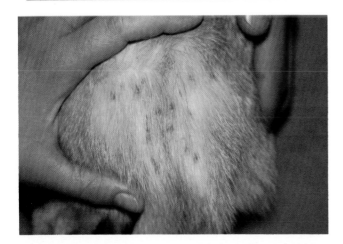

Figure 11-25 *Excoriated papules and self-induced alopecia on dorsal lumbar area of 5-year-old mixed-breed cat. Patient's pruritus and miliary dermatitis were caused by flea bite hypersensitivity.*

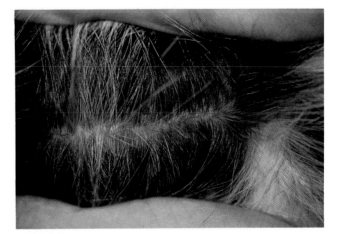

Figure 11-26 *Papules along mid-back of young male cat with miliary dermatitis. Fleas and flea excreta were found at time of examination.*

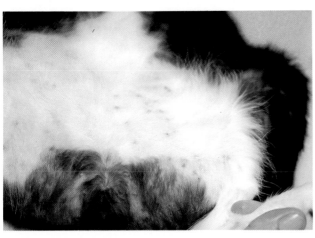

Figure 11-27 *Numerous papules, many of which are excoriated, on abdomen of 6-year-old Domestic Short-Haired cat. Underlying etiology of patient's miliary dermatitis was allergic inhalant disease.*

Neurodermatitis
(Feline Psychogenic Alopecia,
Feline Psychogenic Dermatitis)

CLINICAL SIGNS

1. The most common sign is self-induced hair loss on any part of the body that the cat is able to lick
2. Usually the skin in these involved, alopecic areas is normal
3. In some cases the excessive licking produces erythema, erosions, and excoriated patches

DIFFERENTIAL DIAGNOSIS

1. Flea bite hypersensitivity
2. Food hypersensitivity
3. Allergic inhalant disease (atopy)
4. Dermatophyte infection
5. Demodicosis
6. *Cheyletiella* dermatitis
7. Contact dermatitis
8. Feline "endocrine" alopecia
9. Hyperthyroidism

UNDERLYING ETIOLOGIES

1. Boredom
2. Change in home environment such as a "new" home, new baby, or new owner
3. Stressful home life such as constant arguing by cat owners or change in the day-to-day routine to which cat has become accustomed
4. Acquiring a new pet or losing an existing pet
5. Boarding or hospitalization

DIAGNOSTIC AIDS

1. History may be quite helpful
2. Rule out other differentials for the pruritic cat via skin scraping, dermatophyte culture, fecal flotation, allergy test diet, and intradermal skin testing

COMMENTS

True feline neurodermatitis is an uncommon cause of alopecia in the cat. No age, breed, or sex predilection has been documented. It has been stated that Siamese cats are predisposed. The author believes that neurodermatitis is one of the most *over*diagnosed skin disorders in the cat. Since cats manifest pruritus mainly by licking, great care must be taken to carefully rule out each cause of pruritus before making the diagnosis of "neurodermatitis." The author also believes that most cats diagnosed as having neurodermatitis actually have some form of allergic skin disease.

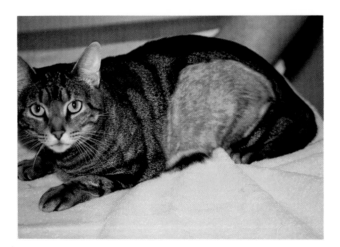

Figure 11-28 Self-induced alopecia on side of 5-year-old Domestic Short-Haired cat. Owners reported that patient licked her side only on weekends when her normal routine was altered.

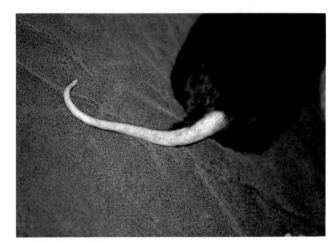

Figure 11-29 Near-total alopecia on tail of Burmese cat. This self-induced disorder was created once a year when cat was boarded for 3 weeks.

Plasma Cell Pododermatitis

CLINICAL SIGNS

1. Swelling and usually subsequent ulceration of the footpad(s)
2. Lesions may be limited to one pad on one foot; however, some cases involve several pads on more than one foot
3. Lesions are mildly to moderately pruritic
4. Pain varies from apparently nonpainful to reluctance to bear weight
5. Some patients also have plasma cell stomatitis

DIFFERENTIAL DIAGNOSIS

1. Neoplasia
2. Eosinophilic plaques
3. Autoimmune and immune-mediated diseases often involve the footpads and/or oral cavity

DIAGNOSTIC AIDS

1. Appearance and location of the lesion(s)
2. Skin biopsies for histopathologic examination show superficial and deep perivascular dermatitis and/or stomatitis with large numbers of plasma cells.

COMMENTS

Plasma cell pododermatitis is rare in the cat. It has not been reported in the dog. No age, breed, or sex predilection exists. The underlying etiology has not been determined.

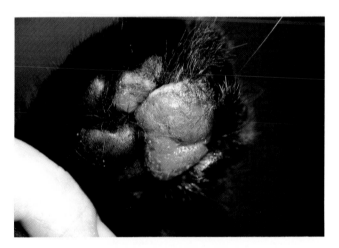

Figure 11-30   *Swollen and ulcerated footpads on forefoot of 3-year-old male mixed Siamese cat with plasma cell pododermatitis. Patient's other feet were not involved.*

Preauricular Alopecia

CLINCIAL SIGNS

1. Varying degrees of alopecia in the preauricular area. (The area between the lateral canthus of the eye and the opening of the external ear canal.)
2. The skin in these areas is normal
3. The patient is not pruritic
4. The alopecic pattern is bilaterally symmetric

DIFFERENTIAL DIAGNOSIS

1. Facial pruritus resulting in self-induced alopecia
2. Demodicosis
3. Dermatophyte infection

COMMENTS

Preauricular alopecia is a common finding in many normal cats. No age, breed, or sex predilections exist. The alopecia is more noticeable in dark-haired cats. Cats are often presented to the veterinarian due to owner concern. However, preauricular alopecia is not a disease and treatment should not be attempted.

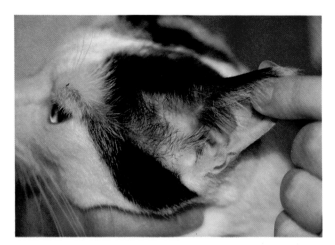

Figure 11-31 *Preauricular alopecia in 11-year-old female spayed cat.*

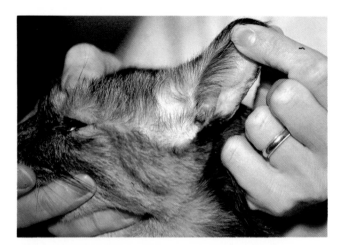

Figure 11-32 *Left preauricular area of 5-year-old female cat shows normal alopecic pattern.*

Self-Induced Alopecia

CLINICAL SIGNS

1. Partial alopecia involving any area of the body that the cat is able to lick
2. Close examination of the alopecic skin reveals short stubbles. (A magnifying loupe is quite helpful.)
3. The skin in involved areas appears normal
4. Alopecic pattern is usually bilaterally symmetric

DIFFERENTIAL DIAGNOSIS
(All causes of non-self-induced alopecia should be considered.)
1. Feline "endocrine" alopecia (rare)
2. Dermatophyte infection
3. Demodicosis

UNDERLYING ETIOLOGIES

1. Allergic inhalant disease
2. Food hypersensitivity
3. Flea bite hypersensitivity
4. Neurodermatitis

5. *Cheyletiella* infestation
6. Pediculosis
7. Intestinal parasitism
8. Dermatophyte infection (may be pruritic)
9. Demodicosis (may also cause self-induced alopecia)

DIAGNOSTIC AIDS

1. A carefully taken history may reveal that the cat is creating the alopecic pattern
2. Microscopic examination of stubbly hairs reveals normal hair bulbs and frayed ends
3. Skin biopsies for histopathologic examination are helpful but usually are not necessary

COMMENTS

Self-induced alopecia is one of the most common presenting signs in feline dermatology. In many cases the owners insist that the alopecia is not created by the cat and is occurring spontaneously. Therefore many cases of self-induced alopecia are misdiagnosed as feline endocrine alopecia, which is quite rare.

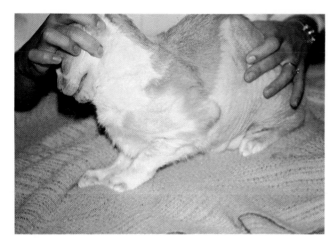

Figure 11-33 Self-induced alopecia on chest, forearms, and entire left side of 6-year-old Domestic Short-Haired cat. Patient's pruritus, which resulted in alopecia, was caused by food hypersensitivity.

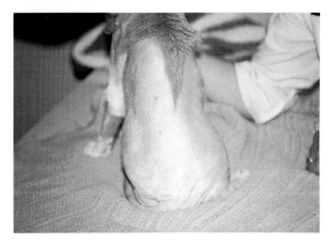

Figure 11-34 Another view of patient shown in Figure 11-33. Areas that this cat is unable to lick have full normal coat.

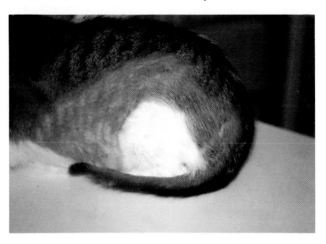

Figure 11-35 Two-year-old female spayed cat shows self-induced alopecia of left side and hip.

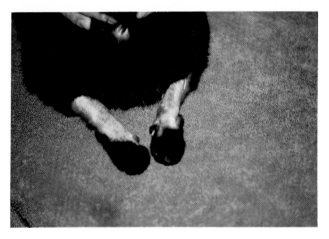

Figure 11-36 *Male altered Domestic Short-Haired cat of unknown age has self-induced alopecia of forelegs. Allergic inhalant disease was cause of this patient's pruritus.*

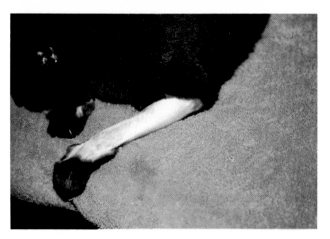

Figure 11-37 *Another view of patient shown in Figure 11-36.*

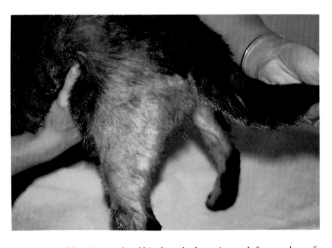

Figure 11-38 *Partial self-induced alopecia on left rear leg of adult male cat. Patient was suffering from flea bite hypersensitivity.*

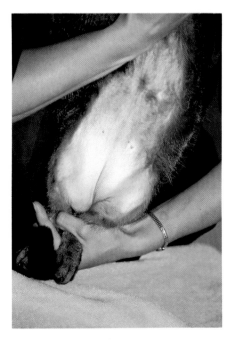

Figure 11-39 *Abdominal area of patient shown in Figure 11-38.*

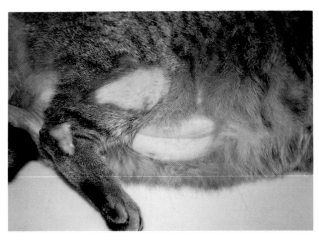

Figure 11-40 *Four-year-old female spayed cat with allergic inhalant disease has self-induced alopecia of right rear leg and abdomen.*

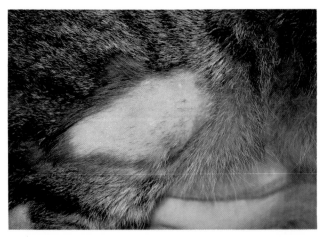

Figure 11-41 *Closer view of alopecic area shown in Figure 11-40.*

TUMORS AND TUMORLIKE LESIONS

Apocrine cyst

Apocrine adenoma (sweat gland adenoma)

Apocrine adenocarcinoma (sweat gland adenocarcinoma)

Basal cell tumor (basal cell carcinoma)

Cutaneous horn

Epidermal inclusion cyst ("sebaceous," epidermal, or epidermoid cyst)

Fibrous histiocytoma (dermatofibroma)

Fibroma (nodular subepidermal fibrosis)

Fibrosarcoma

Hemangioma

Hemangiosarcoma

Hemangiopericytoma (spindle cell sarcoma, dermatofibroma)

Histiocytoma (button tumor)

Cutaneous histiocytosis

Malignant histiocytosis

Keratoacanthoma (intracutaneous cornifying epithelioma)

Lipoma

Cutaneous B-cell lymphosarcoma (nonepitheliotrophic lymphosarcoma)

Cutaneous T-cell lymphosarcoma (mycosis fungoides, epitheliotrophic lymphosarcoma)

Mast cell tumor (mastocytoma)

Benign melanoma (benign dermal melanoma)

Malignant melanoma (malignant dermal melanoma)

Multiple collagenous nevi (idiopathic granulomatous dermatitis, nodular dermatofibrosis)

Neuroendocrine tumor (Merkel cell tumor)

Cutaneous papilloma (wart)

Papillomatosis (oral warts)

Perianal gland tumor (hepatoid gland tumor)

Schwannoma (neurilemoma, neurofibroma)

Nodular sebaceous hyperplasia

Sebaceous adenoma

Sebaceous adenocarcinoma

Skin tag (fibrovascular papilloma, soft fibroma)

Squamous cell carcinoma

Transmissible venereal tumor

Trichoepithelioma

Apocrine Cyst

DESCRIPTION

1. Fluid-filled cystic structures range from 0.5 to 5 cm in diameter
2. Cysts are usually bluish or purplish in color
3. They may be single or muticentric
4. Needle aspirate reveals a clear fluid with no cells

LOCATION

These cysts are most commonly found on the head and neck.

BIOLOGIC BEHAVIOR

Apocrine cysts do not metastasize and do not recur at the surgical site.

COMMENTS

Apocrine cysts are uncommon in the dog and cat. They tend to be multiple in the dog. They are the result of retention of apocrine fluid due to blockage of the excretory duct and are considered to be an aging change.

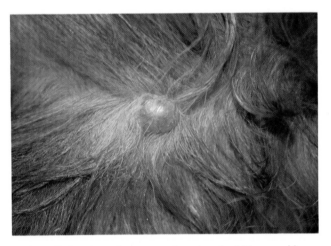

Figure 12-1   *Apocrine cyst on dorsal neck of 11-year-old female spayed Golden Retriever. This lesion was solitary.*

Apocrine Adenoma
(Sweat Gland Adenoma)

DESCRIPTION

1. Apocrine adenomas are firm tumors, but they may have cystic areas
2. They frequently have an ulcerated surface
3. They are usually solitary
4. The tumors may be mutilocular but are relatively well circumscribed
5. Tumors range from 1 to 10 cm in diameter

LOCATION

Tumors may occur anywhere on the skin and in the anal sac walls; however, they may be more common on the back, flanks, and feet.

BIOLOGIC BEHAVIOR

Apocrine adenomas are slow growing. They are rarely invasive and do not metastasize. Surgical excision is curative.

COMMENTS

Apocrine adenomas are relatively uncommon in the dog and cat. No age, breed, or sex predilection has been documented.

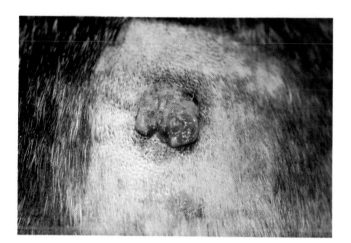

Figure 12-2   *Ulcerated apocrine adenoma on midback of 3-year-old male Bull Mastiff.*

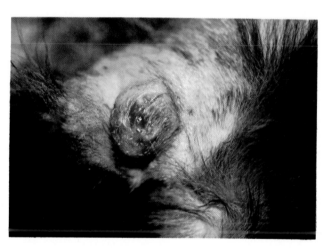

Figure 12-3   *Apocrine cystadenoma with ulcerated surface on head of 9-year-old mixed-breed dog.*

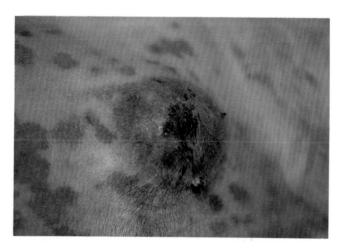

Figure 12-4   *Ulcerated apocrine adenoma measuring 3 × 3 cm on back of 8-year-old male Old English Sheepdog.*

Apocrine Adenocarcinoma (Sweat Gland Adenocarcinoma)

DESCRIPTION

1. Lesions may be solitary and have the same clinical appearance as the apocrine adenomas
2. Some lesions are poorly circumscribed masses that infiltrate large areas of skin and resemble acute moist dermatitis

LOCATION

Tumors may occur anywhere on the skin surface; however, they may be more common in the axillary, inguinal, and perineal areas.

BIOLOGIC BEHAVIOR

Apocrine adenocarcinomas frequently recur at the site of surgical excision. They are often highly invasive and are capable of metastasis to local lymph nodes and the lungs via the lymphatics.

COMMENTS

These carcinomas are uncommon in the dog and cat. No age, breed, or sex predilection has been documented.

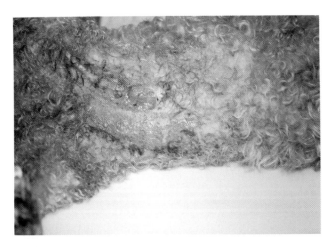

Figure 12-5 *Thirteen-year-old female intact Miniature Poodle with diffuse apocrine adenocarcinoma of abdominal area.*

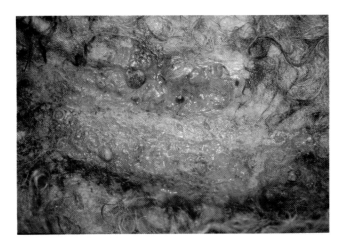

Figure 12-6 *Closer view of patient shown in Figure 12-5.*

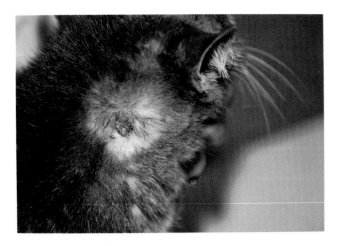

Figure 12-7 *Apocrine adenocarcinoma on neck of 14-year-old female spayed Domestic Short-Haired cat.*

Basal Cell Tumor (Basal Cell Carcinoma)

DESCRIPTION

1. Tumors are solid and elevated, frequently with an ulcerated surface
2. Skin overlying the tumor is usually alopecic
3. Lesions range in size from a few millimeters to several centimeters
4. Most basal cell tumors are solitary; however, they may be multiple

LOCATION

The most common sites of occurrence in the dog are the head, neck, and shoulders. There is no site predilection in the cat.

BIOLOGIC BEHAVIOR

Basal cell tumors are quite benign and rarely recur at the site of surgical excision. They have never been reported to metastasize.

COMMENTS

These tumors are common in the dog and cat between the ages of 8 and 12 years. Poodles and Siamese cats may be predisposed. No sex predilection has been documented.

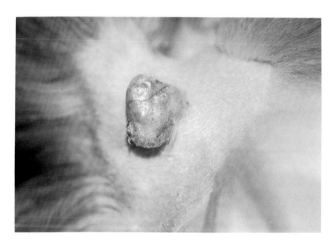

Figure 12-9   *Basal cell tumor, measuring 2 × 3 cm, behind left ear of 11-year-old female spayed Collie.*

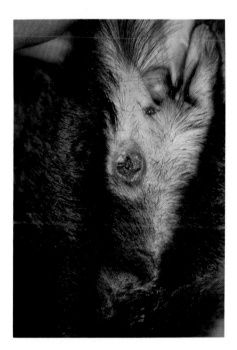

Figure 12-8   *Ulcerated basal cell tumors in preauricular area of male neutered cat of unknown age.*

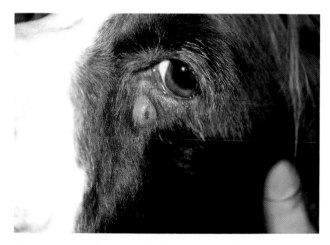

Figure 12-10   *Five-year-old female English Springer Spaniel with solitary facial basal cell tumor.*

Cutaneous Horn

DESCRIPTION

1. Firm, hornlike projections from the skin or footpad surface
2. Horns may be up to 5 cm long
3. Cutaneous horns may be single or multiple

LOCATION

Horns may be located anywhere on the skin surface or footpads.

BIOLOGIC BEHAVIOR

Cutaneous horns are slow growing. The etiology is not known; however, horns have been reported to arise from other keratoses, papillomas, squamous cell carcinomas, and basal cell tumors. The behavior of horns is benign; however, the biologic behavior of the structure from which the horn arose must be considered.

COMMENTS

Cutaneous horns have been reported in dogs and cats. No age, breed, or sex predilection has been reported.

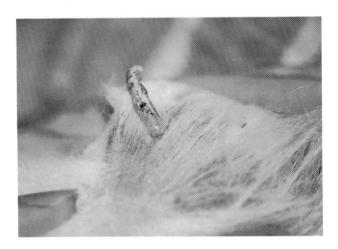

Figure 12-11   *Cutaneous horn on ear pinna of 6-year-old mixed-breed dog.*

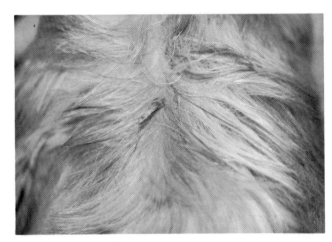

Figure 12-12   *Cutaneous horn (2 cm in length) on midback of 10-year-old female spayed Shih Tzu.*

Epidermal Inclusion Cyst ("Sebaceous", Epidermal, or Epidermoid Cyst)

DESCRIPTION

1. Lesions are solid, smooth, elevated, and round to oval in shape
2. The size of lesions ranges from 0.5 to 4 cm in diameter
3. Epidermal cysts may be single or multiple
4. A tan, grey, or white cheesy material may be expressed from the cysts. This material may also be seen on cut surface.

LOCATION

Epidermal cysts may occur anywhere on the body; however, they are most commonly found on the head, neck, sacral area, and proximal limbs.

BIOLOGIC BEHAVIOR

Epidermal cysts are slow growing and are totally benign. They have never been reported to recur at surgical sites or to metastasize.

COMMENTS

These cysts are common in dogs and uncommon in cats. No age, breed, or sex predilection has been reported.

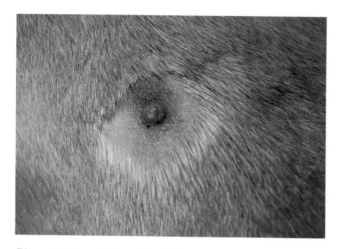

Figure 12-13 *Epidermal inclusion cyst on neck of 4-year-old male English Mastiff.*

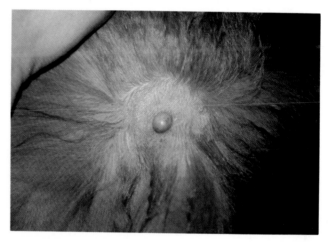

Figure 12-14 *Epidermal inclusion cyst measuring 1 × 1 cm on shoulder of 11-year-old male Shetland Sheepdog.*

Fibrous Histiocytoma (Dermatofibroma)

DESCRIPTION

1. Elevated, firm, plaquelike lesions
2. Size ranges from 0.5 to several centimeters in diameter
3. Lesions are usually solitary but may be multiple
4. The surface is usually alopecic and may be ulcerated

LOCATION

Lesions most frequently occur on the face; however, any area of the body may be involved.

BIOLOGIC BEHAVIOR

Fibrous histiocytomas are locally invasive. They frequently recur at the site of surgical excision but rarely metastasize.

COMMENTS

Fibrous histiocytomas are uncommon in dogs and rare in cats. They differ from "typical" histiocytomas not only in their histopathologic appearance but also in their biologic behavior. These tumors may be more common in Collies and in dogs between 2 and 4 years of age.

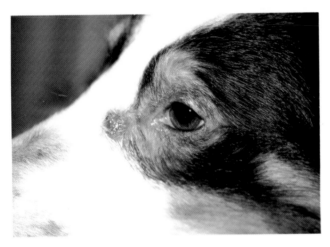

Figure 12-15   *Fibrous histiocytoma near medial canthus of left eye of 2-year-old Shetland Sheepdog. (Periocular self-induced alopecia and erythema are also evident.)*

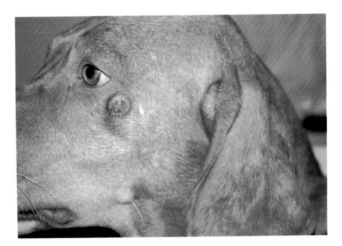

Figure 12-16   *Buttonlike ulcerated fibrous histiocytoma on face of young male Vizsla.*

Fibroma
(Nodular Subepidermal Fibrosis)

DESCRIPTION

1. Fibromas may be firm or soft
2. They may be pedunculated or dome shaped
3. These tumors are located in the dermis or subcutis and are firmly attached to the overlying epidermis
4. The tumor surface may be devoid of hair but rarely is ulcerated
5. Fibromas are usually solitary, but they may be multiple

LOCATION

The limbs, flanks, and groin appear to be the most common sites of occurrence of fibromas in the dog.

BIOLOGIC BEHAVIOR

Fibromas do not metastasize and rarely recur at the site of excision.

COMMENTS

Fibromas are uncommon in the dog and cat. Older animals are predisposed. No sex or breed predilection has been documented.

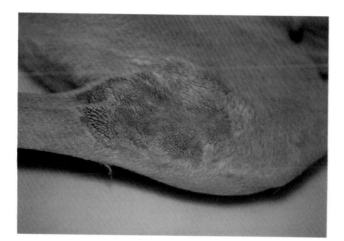

Figure 12-17　Nodular subepidermal fibrosis on medial aspect of right rear leg of young female dog.

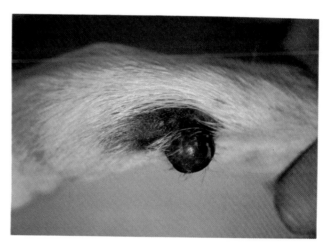

Figure 12-18　Pigmented, pedunculated fibroma on foreleg of 9-year-old male mixed-breed dog.

Fibrosarcoma

DESCRIPTION

1. Tumor consistency may be firm or fleshy
2. The tumor is closely attached to surrounding tissues
3. The surface is usually ulcerated
4. Fibrosarcomas are usually solitary in the dog

LOCATION

The most common locations are the limbs and trunk. Fibrosarcoma is the second most common intraoral malignancy in the dog.

BIOLOGIC BEHAVIOR

Fibrosarcomas are rapidly growing and invasive. In approximately 30% of cases there is local recurrence, and in 10% of cases metastasis occurs.

COMMENTS

Fibrosarcomas are uncommon in the dog and cat. No age, breed, or sex predilection has been documented. Some cases of feline fibrosarcoma are virus induced and usually occur in young animals. The virus, feline sarcoma virus, is closely related to feline leukemia virus, and cats with multiple cutaneous fibrosarcomas are feline leukemia virus-positive.

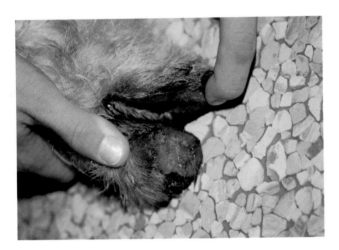

Figure 12-19   *Ulcerated digital fibrosarcoma in 3-year-old Irish Wolfhound.*

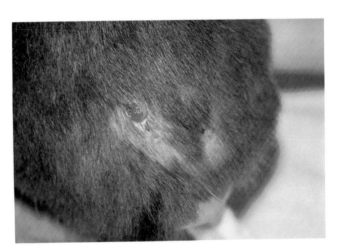

Figure 12-20   *Multiple fibrosarcomas on rump of cat. This patient tested positive for feline leukemia virus.*

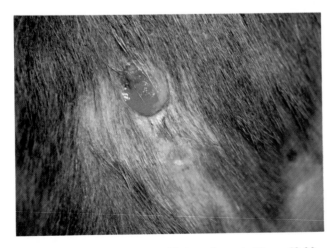

Figure 12-21   *Closer view of lesions shown in Figure 12-20.*

Hemangioma

DESCRIPTION

1. Hemangiomas are firm to fluctuant and are well circumscribed
2. They are typically round to oval and color is bluish, purplish, or black
3. Hemangiomas are usually solitary
4. Lesions range in size from 0.5 to 4 cm

LOCATION

Hemangiomas may be located anywhere on the body, but the neck, face, limbs, and flanks are sites of predilection.

BIOLOGIC BEHAVIOR

Hemangiomas are benign. They rarely recur at the site of surgical excision and do not metastasize.

COMMENTS

Hemangiomas are rare in cats and common in dogs. No breed or sex predilection has been documented. Older animals are predisposed.

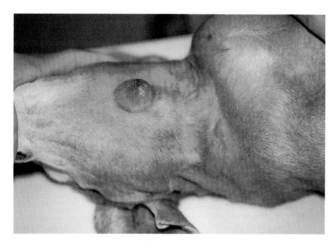

Figure 12-22   Hemangioma on ventral neck area of 11-year-old Short-Haired Dachshund. (Area has been cleaned with iodine solution.)

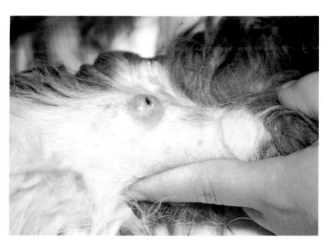

Figure 12-23   Right foreleg of 8-year-old Old English Sheepdog has 1.5 × 1 cm purplish mass. Small area of central ulceration can be seen.

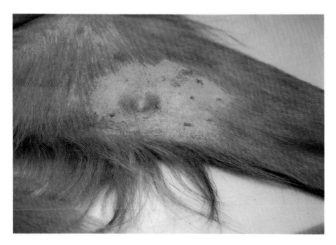

Figure 12-24   Right rear leg of female Irish Setter has 2 × 1 cm blue-black hemangioma.

Hemangiosarcoma

DESCRIPTION

1. Lesions are usually nodular or dome shaped
2. The color varies from blue to purple to black
3. Tumors range from a few millimeters to several centimeters in diameter
4. Hemangiosarcomas are rarely ulcerated
5. Tumors may be solitary or multiple

LOCATION

Lesions may arise anywhere; however, they may occur more frequently on the extremities and abdomen.

BIOLOGIC BEHAVIOR

Hemangiosarcomas are highly invasive and have a very high rate of metastasis. Cutaneous hemangiosarcomas may be the metastatic lesions of internal hemangiosarcomas, especially splenic ones.

COMMENTS

Hemangiosarcomas are uncommon to rare neoplasms of the dog and cat. Older animals are predisposed. Canine breed predispositions include German Shepherd Dogs, Boxers, Collies, and Golden Retrievers. Male dogs appear to be predisposed. No breed and sex predilections have been documented in the cat.

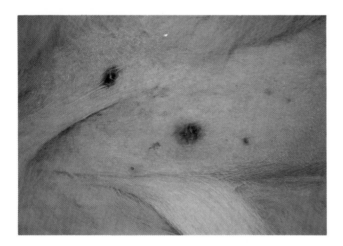

Figure 12-25 *Abdomen of 12-year-old female spayed Shetland Sheepdog with multiple cutaneous hemangiosarcomas, apparently arising from splenic hemangiosarcoma.*

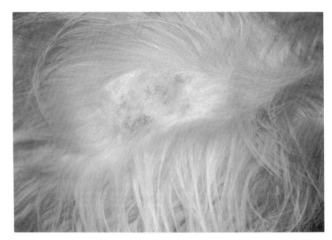

Figure 12-26 *Hemangiosarcoma on right flank of 10-year-old male Golden Retriever.*

Hemangiopericytoma (Spindle Cell Sarcoma, Dermatofibroma)

DESCRIPTION

1. Hemangiopericytomas are firm, elevated masses located intradermally and subcutaneously
2. The tumor surface may be devoid of hair
3. Occasionally the surface will ulcerate
4. Tumors are usually solitary
5. Tumors range in size from 2 to 25 cm

LOCATION

The most common location is the limbs, especially over joints. Tumors also occur on the thorax and ventral abdomen.

BIOLOGIC BEHAVIOR

Hemangiopericytomas are exceedingly infiltrative. More than 30% are reported to recur at the site of surgical excision. Radiation therapy may increase the tendency for recurrence. The tumors almost never metastasize.

COMMENTS

Hemangiopericytomas are rare in cats and common in dogs. Older dogs and female animals are predisposed. Several canine breed predilections have been reported, including German Shepherd Dogs, Labrador Retrievers, Golden Retrievers, Boxers, Cocker and Springer Spaniels.

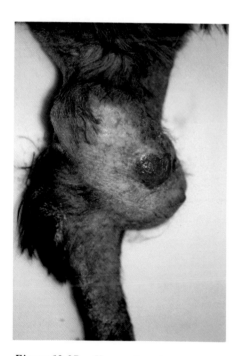

Figure 12-27 *Hemangiopericytoma on rear leg of 13-year-old Cocker Spaniel.*

Histiocytoma (Button Tumor)

DESCRIPTION

1. Histiocytomas are elevated, somewhat firm, and dome shaped
2. Most tumors are quite erythematous
3. The surface is usually devoid of hair and may be ulcerated
4. Most tumors are solitary
5. They range in diameter from 0.5 to 3 cm

LOCATION

The head, ear pinnae, and limbs are the most commonly involved sites. The tumor, however, may occur anywhere on the body.

BIOLOGIC BEHAVIOR

Histiocytomas are benign. They neither metastasize nor do they recur at the site of surgical excision. Most tumors spontaneously regress within a few months.

COMMENTS

Histiocytomas are very common in the dog and rare in the cat. These tumors occur most frequently in dogs under 2 years of age. No breed or sex predilection has been documented.

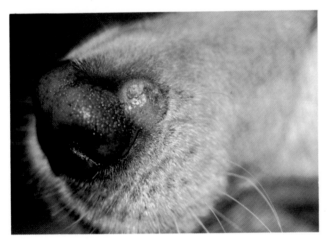

Figure 12-28 *Histiocytoma on muzzle of 18-month-old Labrador Retriever.*

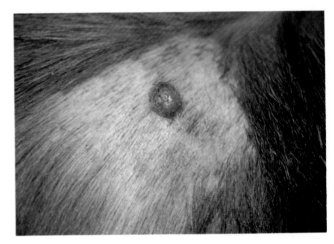

Figure 12-29 *Histiocytoma on right shoulder of young Shetland Sheepdog.*

Cutaneous Histiocytosis

DESCRIPTION

1. Multiple, firm nodules or plaques that frequently coalesce
2. The surface is usually alopecic and erythematous
3. Pruritus is mild to nonexistent
4. Size of lesions may range from 1 to 7 cm

LOCATION

No sites of predilection have been reported. Lesions may occur anywhere on the body.

BIOLOGIC BEHAVIOR

Cutaneous histiocytosis is considered to be benign. Metastasis has never been reported, but lesions are difficult to surgically excise and frequently recur at the site of excision.

COMMENTS

Cutaneous histiocytosis is a rare disease of the dog and cat. No age, breed, or sex predilection has been reported.

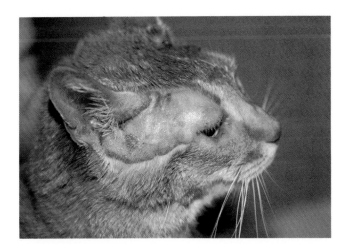

Figure 12-30   *Cutaneous histiocytosis of periocular and preauricular areas of 8-year-old male Domestic Short-Haired cat.*

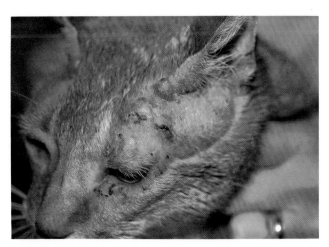

Figure 12-31   *Left side of face of patient shown in Figure 12-30. This patient's cutaneous histiocytosis was strikingly bilaterally symmetric.*

Malignant Histiocytosis

DESCRIPTION

1. Lesions consist of multiple cutaneous plaques or nodules that may coalesce
2. Lesions may be alopecic, erythematous, or ulcerated
3. Pruritus may be significant
4. Lesions vary greatly in size but may be up to 10 cm in diameter

LOCATION

No sites of predilection have been reported. Lesions may occur anywhere on the body.

BIOLOGIC BEHAVIOR

Cutaneous lesions are usually associated with signs of systemic illness, including peripheral lymphadenopathy, hepatomegaly, splenomegaly, lethargy, anorexia, and weight loss. The disease is considered to be highly malignant.

COMMENTS

Malignant histiocytosis is a rare disease of dogs. Male Bernese Mountain Dogs may be predisposed.

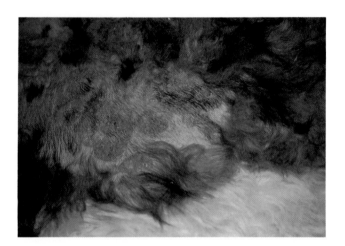

Figure 12-32 *Five-year-old male Old English Sheepdog with malignant histiocytosis. This patient's entire trunk was covered with coalescing, erythematous, targetlike plaques.*

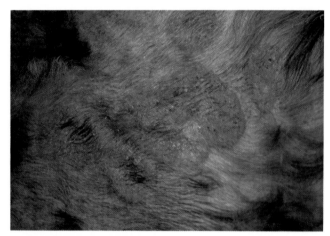

Figure 12-33 *Closer view of lesions from patient shown in Figure 12-32.*

Keratoacanthoma (Intracutaneous Cornifying Epithelioma)

DESCRIPTION

1. Keratoacanthomas are firm to fluctuant masses in the dermis or subcutis
2. These tumors have a visible opening or pore in the center. The pore contains a plug of keratin material
3. Tumors may be solitary or multiple
4. Tumors range in diameter from 0.5 to 4 cm

LOCATION

Keratoacanthomas are most frequently located on the trunk, but any area on the body may be involved.

BIOLOGIC BEHAVIOR

Tumors are slow growing and benign. They frequently become ulcerated and secondarily infected with bacteria. Because of the size and number of these tumors in some patients, surgical excision may be quite difficult.

COMMENTS

Keratoacanthomas are common tumors of the dog. They have not been documented in the cat. Multiple keratoacanthomas are more common in certain breeds of dogs including the Keeshond and Norwegian Elkhound. Male dogs less than 5 years of age appear to be predisposed.

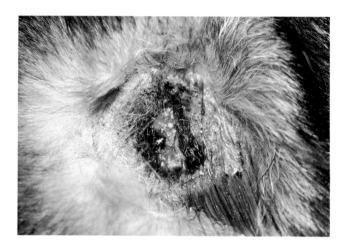

Figure 12-34   *Ulcerated, infected keratoacanthoma on lateral thorax of 7-year-old male Norwegian Elkhound.*

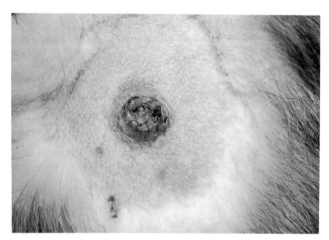

Figure 12-35   *Another keratoacanthoma on trunk of patient shown in Figure 12-34.*

Lipoma

DESCRIPTION

1. Most lipomas are oval or dome shaped
2. They are subcutaneous in location
3. Most lipomas are soft, but they may be firm due to fibrous connective tissue infiltration
4. Most are movable over the underlying tissues
5. Lipomas range from 1 to 25 cm in diameter

LOCATION

Most lipomas are found on the thorax, abdomen, and rear limbs; however, they may occur anywhere on the body.

BIOLOGIC BEHAVIOR

Typical lipomas do not recur at the site of surgical excision and do not metastasize. Infiltrative lipomas and liposarcomas frequently recur at the site of surgical excision.

COMMENTS

Lipomas are common benign neoplasms of the dog. They are less common in the cat. The age of affected dogs ranges from 2 to 18 years, with a peak incidence between 8 and 12 years. Females and obese animals are predisposed.

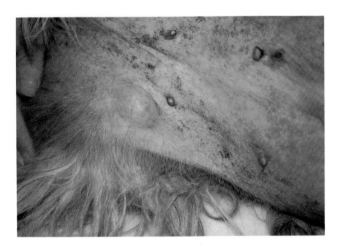

Figure 12-36 *Lipoma in inguinal area of middle-aged female Lhasa Apso.*

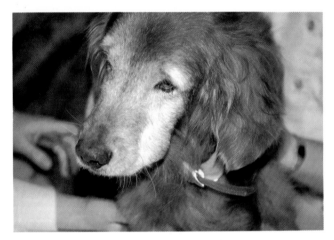

Figure 12-37 *Lipoma on left side of face of 12-year-old Golden Retriever.*

Cutaneous B-Cell Lymphosarcoma (Nonepitheliotrophic Lymphosarcoma)

DESCRIPTION

1. Cutaneous lesions may appear as any of the following: ulcers, nodules, plaques, pustules, erythroderma, and exfoliative dermatitis
2. Lesions are typically multifocal or generalized
3. Peripheral lymphadenopathy may be present
4. Signs of other organ involvement may be present
5. Pruritus is variable

LOCATION

There is no site predilection. Any area of the trunk, head, or limbs may be involved.

BIOLOGIC BEHAVIOR

Cutaneous lymphosarcoma is a highly malignant disease. Surgical excision is usually impractical because of the large numbers of lesions. When surgical excision is attempted, recurrence is common. This neoplastic disease metastasizes to the lymph nodes, liver, lung, spleen, and other internal organs. The disease is usually fatal within 6 months of diagnosis.

COMMENTS

Cutaneous lymphosarcoma is an uncommon or rare disease of the dog and cat. Animals over 8 years of age appear to be predisposed. No breed or sex predilection has been documented. In cats this disease is associated with the feline leukemia virus even though affected cats may test feline leukemia virus-negative.

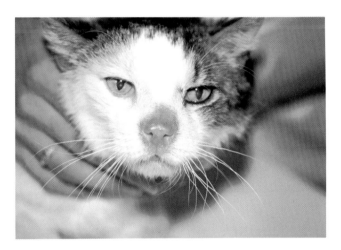

Figure 12-38 *Cutaneous lymphosarcoma involving nose of 17-year-old male Domestic Short-Haired cat.*

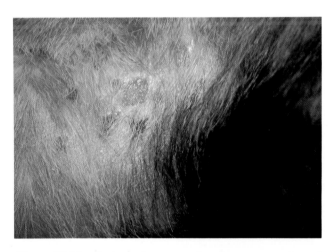

Figure 12-39 *Lesions of cutaneous lymphosarcoma on lateral thoracic area of 15-year-old female Calico cat.*

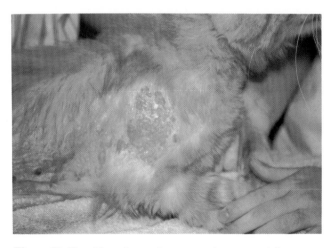

Figure 12-40 *Alopecic, erythematous plaques on right shoulder and lateral thoracic areas of 10-year-old male Domestic Short-Haired cat.*

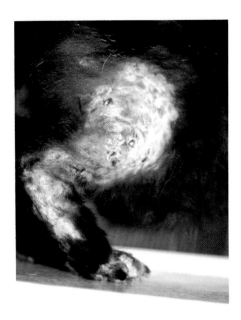

Figure 12-41 *Alopecia, erythema, ulcerated plaques, and scaling on right rear leg of 18-year-old female cat.*

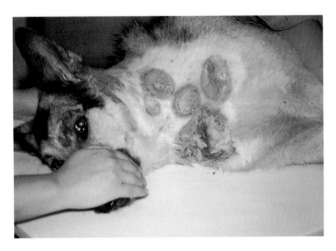

Figure 12-42 *Numerous circular and ringlike ulcerated plaques on face, neck, and shoulders of 9-year-old male German Shepherd Dog with lymphosarcoma.*

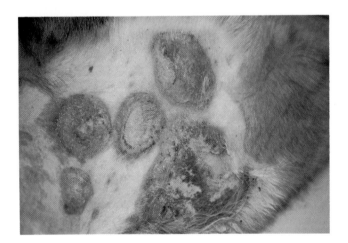

Figure 12-43 *Closer view of lesions shown in Figure 12-42.*

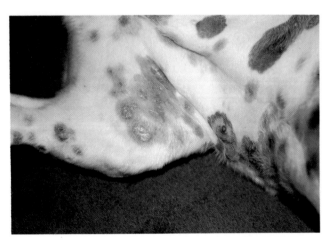

Figure 12-44 *Three-year-old female mixed Dalmatian with numerous, coalescing, erythematous, ulcerated plaques on abdomen and rear leg.*

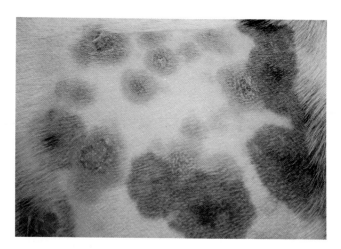

Figure 12-45   *Closer view of lesions from patient shown in Figure 12-44.*

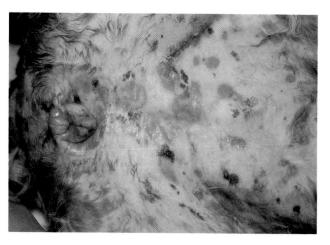

Figure 12-46   *Ulcerated plaquelike lesions on abdomen and vulva of 10-year-old English Cocker Spaniel with cutaneous lymphosarcoma.*

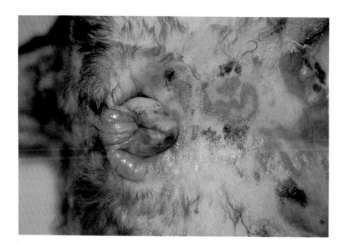

Figure 12-47   *Closer view of lesions shown in Figure 12-46.*

Cutaneous T-Cell Lymphosarcoma (Mycosis Fungoides, Epitheliotrophic Lymphosarcoma)

DESCRIPTION

1. Several clinical presentations have been recognized. These include generalized exfoliative dermatitis— alopecia, erythema, and fine to coarse white scales; swelling and erythema with hypopigmentation or depigmentation of the nose, lips, eyelids, prepuce, or vulva; and ulcerative oral cavity disease.
2. Pruritus is variable

LOCATION

Any area of the body may be involved, but the mucocutaneous junctions and oral cavity are sites of predilection.

BIOLOGIC BEHAVIOR

T-cell lymphosarcoma is a highly malignant disease. Metastasis to lymph nodes and internal organs, especially the gastrointestinal system, is common. Death usually occurs within 4 to 8 months of diagnosis.

COMMENTS

T-cell lymphosarcoma is an uncommon neoplastic disease of the dog and cat. No sex or breed predilection has been reported. Older animals are predisposed.

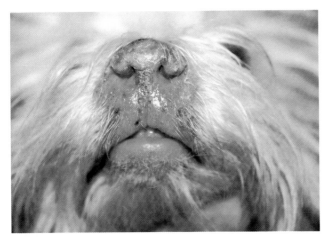

Figure 12-48   *Cutaneous lymphosarcoma in 13-year-old West Highland White Terrier. This patient's puffy and erythematous lips, nasal philtrum, and nose are classic presentation.*

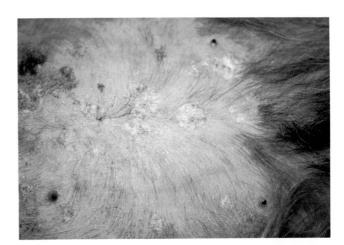

Figure 12-49   *Scaley white, erythematous plaques on abdomen of 6-year-old Cairn Terrier.*

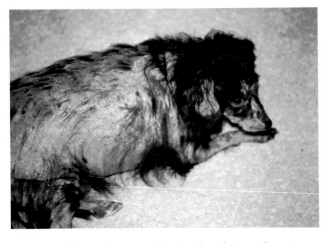

Figure 12-50   *Twelve-year-old mixed-breed dog with severe, generalized cutaneous lymphosarcoma.*

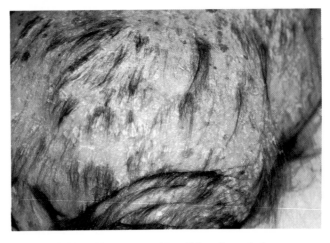

Figure 12-51   *Closer view of T-cell lymphoma lesions on patient shown in Figure 12-50.*

Mast Cell Tumor (Mastocytoma)

DESCRIPTION

1. The clinical appearance of mast cell tumors varies greatly
2. Tumors are round to oval in shape and they may coalesce
3. Most mast cell tumors are firm, but they may be spongy or edematous
4. The surface is usually alopecic and erythematous
5. The surface may be ulcerated
6. Mast cell tumors may be single or multiple
7. Tumors range in diameter from 1 to greater than 10 cm

LOCATION

Canine mast cell tumors occur most frequently on limbs, trunk, and perineum. In cats the head and neck are sites of predilection for mast cell tumors.

BIOLOGIC BEHAVIOR

The biologic behavior of mast cell tumors varies greatly. Some tumors are solitary benign masses that are easily surgically excised and do not recur at the site of excision. Others are highly malignant and metastasize rapidly.

COMMENTS

Mast cell tumors are common neoplasms of the dog and cat. These tumors occur at any age in dogs, with no sex predilection. Some breeds are predisposed, including Boston Terriers, Boxers, and Weimaraners. In cats adult males appear to be predisposed.

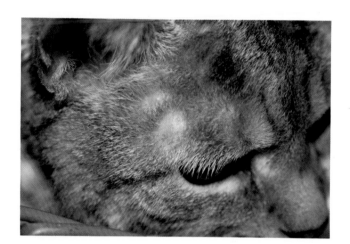

Figure 12-52   *Alopecic, slightly erythematous, nodular lesions in preauricular area of Domestic Short-Haired cat.*

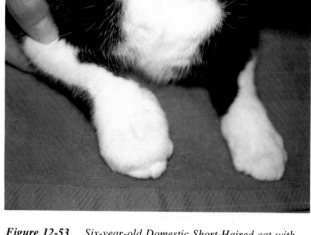

Figure 12-53   *Six-year-old Domestic Short-Haired cat with markedly swollen right distal foreleg. This entire swelling was malignant mast cell tumor.*

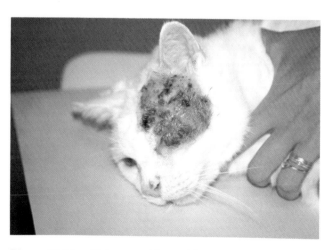

Figure 12-54   *Eight-year-old cat with extensive, ulcerated, highly malignant mast cell tumor on face.*

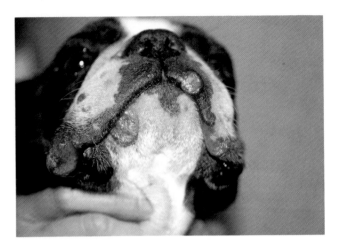

Figure 12-55 *Several ulcerated mast cell tumors on lips of 6-year-old Boston Terrier.*

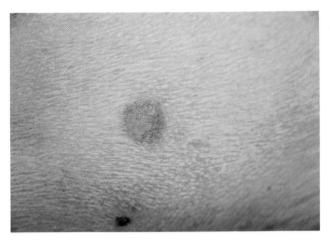

Figure 12-56 *Mast cell tumor on lateral thorax of 8-year-old Boxer. This patient had numerous cutaneous mast cell tumors.*

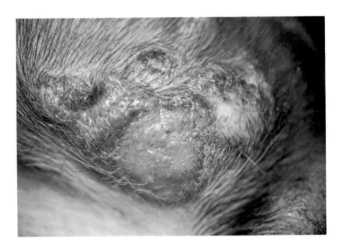

Figure 12-57 *Grouped, ulcerated mast cell tumors on medial thigh of 10-year-old male Boston Terrier.*

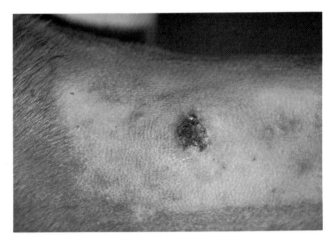

Figure 12-58 *Ulcerated mast cell tumor on rear leg of 3-year-old Boxer. (Surrounding lesions are bacterial folliculitis.)*

Benign Melanoma (Benign Dermal Melanoma)

DESCRIPTION

1. Lesions range in color from light brown to black
2. Lesions may be macules or firm, raised nodules
3. The surface of most benign melanomas is not alopecic or ulcerated
4. Most melanomas are solitary
5. Size of lesions range from 0.25 to 3 cm

LOCATION

Benign dermal melanomas are most frequently found on the head, eyelids, and forelimbs in dogs. There are no reported sites of predilection for benign melanomas in cats.

BIOLOGIC BEHAVIOR

Benign dermal melanomas do not metastasize and do not recur at the site of surgical excision.

COMMENTS

Benign melanomas are common in the dog and rare in the cat. No age or sex predilection has been documented. Certain breeds of dogs appear to be predisposed. These include Scottish Terriers, Schnauzers, Irish Setters, and Doberman Pinschers. No breed predilections have been reported in the cat.

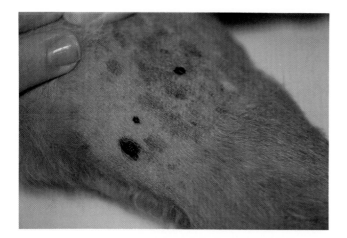

Figure 12-59 *Three benign melanomas on rear leg of young Chesapeake Bay Retriever.*

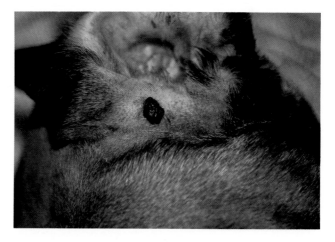

Figure 12-60 *Benign melanoma in preauricular area of 4-year-old Bull Mastiff.*

Malignant Melanoma
(Malignant Dermal Melanoma)

DESCRIPTION

1. Malignant melanomas are often less pigmented than benign melanomas
2. Malignant melanomas may be totally lacking in pigment
3. Lesions consist of raised plaques or nodules
4. The surface is alopecic and ulceration is common
5. The tumor size varies but is usually greater than 2 cm in diameter

LOCATION

In dogs malignant melanomas are most frequently located at the mucocutaneous junction of the lips and on the digits. In cats the face and ear pinnae are sites of predilection.

BIOLOGIC BEHAVIOR

Malignant melanomas frequently recur at the site of surgical excision and frequently metastasize to local lymph nodes and the lungs.

COMMENTS

Malignant melanomas are less common in the dog than are benign melanomas. In the cat most dermal melanomas are malignant. Several breeds of dogs have been reported to be at increased risk for developing these tumors. In cats no breed predilection exists. The age of affected animals varies greatly.

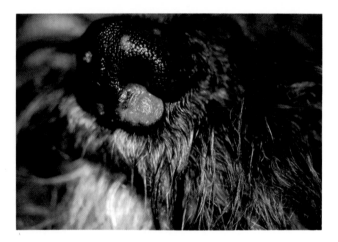

Figure 12-61 *Ulcerated malignant melanoma on nose of 9-year-old male Scottish Terrier.*

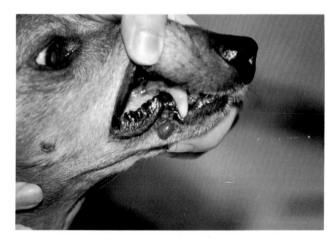

Figure 12-62 *Malignant melanoma on lower lip of 14-year-old Dachshund.*

Multiple Collagenous Nevi (Idiopathic Granulomatous Dermatitis, Nodular Dermatofibrosis)

DESCRIPTION

1. Multiple, firm, asymptomatic nodules in the skin
2. The nodules are usually covered by normal-appearing skin and haircoat; however, they may be alopecic and may have a dimpled surface
3. Nodules range in diameter from 0.4 to 3.5 cm

LOCATION

The most common areas of involvement are the distal limbs and face; however, any area of the body may be involved.

BIOLOGIC BEHAVIOR

The lesions are considered to be benign, but surgical removal is almost impossible due to the high numbers of nodules in most patients. In German Shepherd Dogs the nevi are usually associated with renal cystadenocarcinoma and/or uterine leiomyomas.

COMMENTS

Multiple collagenous nevi have been reported in several breeds of dogs. The disease has not been reported in cats. German Shepherd Dogs appear to be predisposed. No age or sex predilection has been documented.

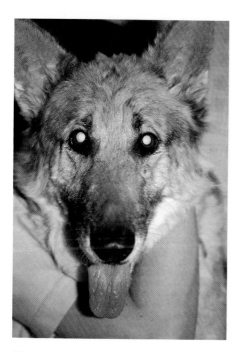

Figure 12-63   *Nine-year-old German Shepherd Dog with multiple collagenous nevi has "lumpy-bumpy" appearance of face and head.*

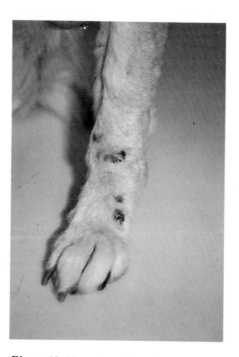

Figure 12-64   *Several hyperpigmented nodules on distal foreleg of patient shown in Figure 12-63.*

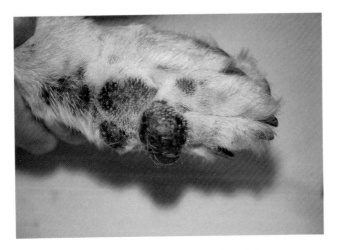

Figure 12-65 *Numerous, hyperpigmented nodules, some ulcerated, on left rear foot of patient shown in Figures 12-63 and 12-64.*

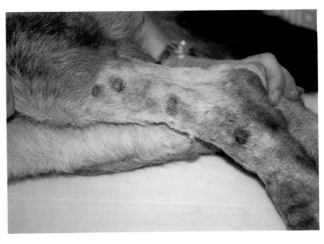

Figure 12-66 *Left rear leg of 4-year-old German Shepherd Dog has several hyperpigmented multiple collagenous nevi.*

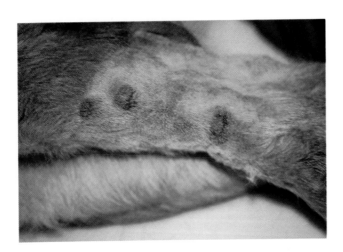

Figure 12-67 *Closer view of lesions shown in Figure 12-66. (Hair has been shaved from involved area.)*

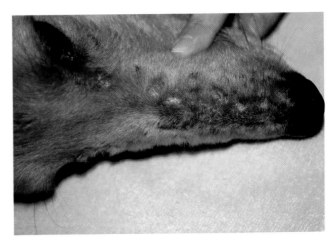

Figure 12-68 *Face of middle-aged Collie with multiple collagenous nevi. This patient's cutaneous disease was not associated with renal disease.*

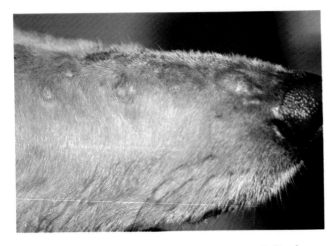

Figure 12-69 *Another view of facial lesions on Collie shown in Figure 12-68. Nevi were also present on ear pinnae and distal extremities.*

Neuroendocrine Tumor (Merkel Cell Tumor)

DESCRIPTION

1. Neuroendocrine tumors are elevated, firm nodules
2. The surface is usually alopecic but rarely ulcerated
3. These tumors are usually solitary but may be multiple
4. Tumors range in diameter from 1 to 3 cm

LOCATION

The most common sites of occurrence are the lips, ears, digits, and mucocutaneous junctions. These tumors may occur in the oral cavity.

BIOLOGIC BEHAVIOR

Neuroendocrine tumors rarely recur at the site of surgical excision. There have, however, been rare reports of metastasis.

COMMENTS

Neuroendocrine tumors are uncommon in the dog. They have not been reported in the cat. No breed or sex predilection has been documented. Affected dogs range in age from 3 to 15 years.

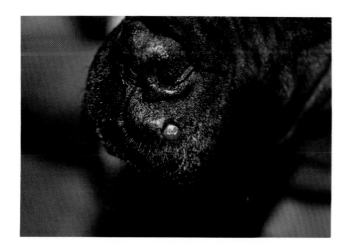

Figure 12-70   *Neuroendocrine tumor on muzzle of 9-year-old Bull Mastiff.*

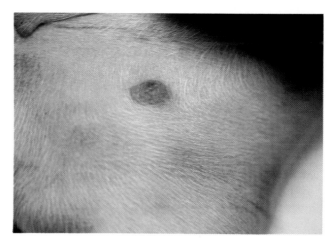

Figure 12-71   *Elevated erythematous lesion on medial thigh of 8-year-old mixed Beagle.*

Cutaneous Papilloma (Wart)

DESCRIPTION

1. Most papillomas are cauliflower like or pedunculated
2. The surface is alopecic and occasionally is ulcerated
3. Lesions may be single or multiple
4. Papillomas are usually less than 0.5 cm in diameter

LOCATION

Papillomas may be located anywhere on the body; however, sites of predilection include the head, eyelids, and feet.

BIOLOGIC BEHAVIOR

Papillomas are considered to be benign. In some cases cutaneous papillomas are virus induced. They rarely have been reported to develop into squamous cell carcinomas.

COMMENTS

Papillomas are very common in the dog and rare in the cat. Older animals are predisposed. No breed or sex predilection exists in the cat. Male dogs, Cocker Spaniels, and Poodles may be predisposed.

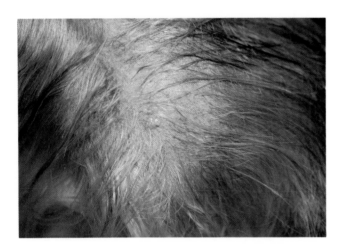

Figure 12-72   *Small, yellowish papilloma on back of 11-year-old Shih Tzu.*

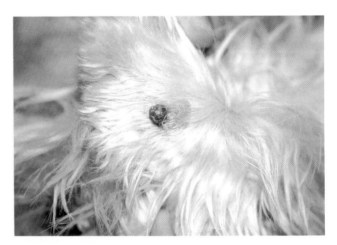

Figure 12-73   *Pigmented papilloma on ear pinna of 14-year-old West Highland White Terrier.*

Papillomatosis (Oral Warts)

DESCRIPTION

1. Lesions are multiple and usually grouped or coalescing
2. The surface of lesions may be smooth or cauliflower like
3. The color varies from white to tan to grey
4. Lesions do not appear to be painful nor pruritic, but they may bleed with mild trauma such as normal chewing
5. Size of lesions varies from less than 1 cm to several centimeters in diameter

LOCATION

Lesions are commonly located on the lips, buccal mucosa, tongue, hard palate, soft palate, and pharynx.

BIOLOGIC BEHAVIOR

Oral papillomatosis is virus induced and contagious to other dogs. Lesions do not metastasize and often spontaneously regress.

COMMENTS

Oral papillomatosis is uncommon in dogs. It has not been reported in the cat. Young dogs are predisposed. No breed or sex predilection has been reported.

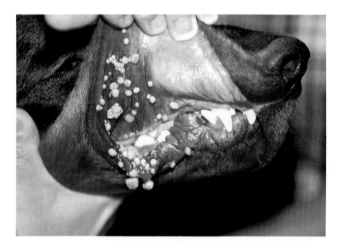

Figure 12-74   *Extensive oral papillomatosis in 7-month-old Doberman Pinscher.*

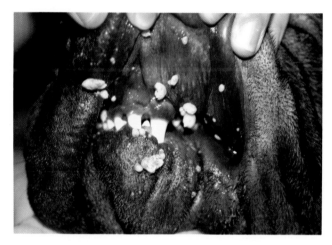

Figure 12-75   *Numerous oral papillomatosis lesions in 4-month-old Chinese Shar Pei.*

Perianal Gland Tumor (Hepatoid Gland Tumor)

DESCRIPTION

1. Lesions are oval or round in shape and they may be multinodular
2. They are raised and rubbery and may be well circumscribed
3. Ulceration and secondary bacterial infection are common
4. Tumors may be solitary or multiple
5. Tumor size may range from less than 1 cm to several centimeters in diameter

LOCATION

The most common location for perianal gland tumors is around the anus. These tumors also may be found on the tail, prepuce, perineum, rump, and thigh.

BIOLOGIC BEHAVIOR

Hepatoid gland tumors may be classified as hyperplasia, adenoma, or adenocarcinoma. Hyperplastic lesions and adenomas are benign. Adenocarcinomas grow rapidly, are infiltrative, and frequently metastasize.

COMMENTS

Perianal gland (hepatoid) tumors are common in the dog. Older dogs and males are predisposed. Growth of perianal gland hyperplasia and perianal gland adenomas is influenced by sex hormones. Other tumors affecting the perianal area may arise from modified apocrine glands.

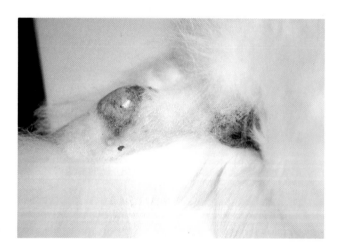

Figure 12-76   *Hepatoid gland tumor on tail of 11-year-old male intact Samoyed. Tumor measured 3 × 4 cm.*

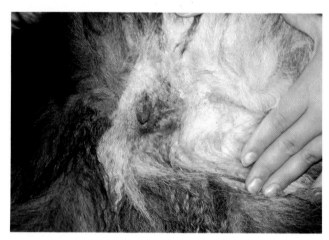

Figure 12-77   *Ulcerated hepatoid gland tumor in perianal area of 14-year-old male intact mixed-breed dog.*

Schwannoma
(Neurilemoma, Neurofibroma)

DESCRIPTION

1. Schwannomas are firm tumors that are usually solitary
2. They may be well or poorly circumscribed
3. The tumor surface may be ulcerated
4. Size varies greatly

LOCATION

In cats the tumors are most frequently located on the head and neck. In dogs the limbs are sites of predilection.

BIOLOGIC BEHAVIOR

In cats schwannomas are frequently malignant. In dogs these tumors are usually benign.

COMMENTS

Schwannomas are rare in the dog and cat. They usually occur in older animals. No breed or sex predilection has been documented.

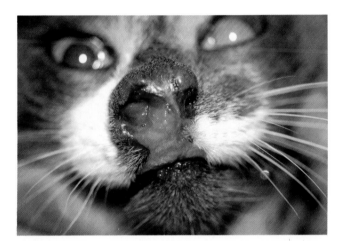

Figure 12-78 *Ulcerated invasive malignant schwannoma on nose and lip of 14-year-old female Domestic Short-Haired cat.*

Nodular Sebaceous Hyperplasia

DESCRIPTION

1. Lesions are firm and elevated
2. The surface is devoid of hair and may be shiny and/ or cauliflower like
3. Occasionally the surface is ulcerated
4. Color of lesions ranges from pink to yellow
5. Lesions are multiple
6. Most lesions are less than 1 cm in diameter

LOCATION

Nodular sebaceous hyperplasia may occur anywhere on the body.

BIOLOGIC BEHAVIOR

Nodular sebaceous hyperplasia is benign; however, surgical excision may be quite frustrating due to the large numbers of lesions in many patients.

COMMENTS

Sebaceous gland hyperplasia is very common in dogs and rare in cats. It is the most common sebaceous gland tumor in both species. Older animals are predisposed. No sex predisposition has been reported. Predisposed canine breeds include Cocker Spaniels, Poodles, and Dachshunds.

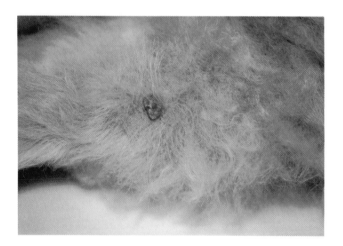

Figure 12-79 *Nodular sebaceous hyperplasia on flank of 9-year-old Cocker-Poodle cross.*

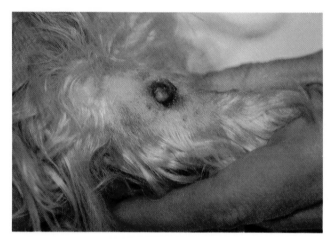

Figure 12-80 *Nodular sebaceous hyperplasia on foreleg of 13-year-old mixed Poodle.*

Sebaceous Adenoma

DESCRIPTION

1. Sebaceous adenomas are usually larger (up to 2 cm in diameter) than sebaceous hyperplasia lesions
2. Lesions are firm and well circumscribed and usually are easily movable over underlying tissues
3. The surface of lesions is frequently alopecic and may be ulcerated
4. Tumors may be solitary or multiple

LOCATION

Any area of the body may be involved, but the head, abdomen, and thorax appear to be sites of predilection.

BIOLOGIC BEHAVIOR

Sebaceous adenomas are benign. They do not recur at the site of surgical excision and do not metastasize.

COMMENTS

Sebaceous adenomas are very common in the dog and rare in the cat. Older dogs are predisposed. These tumors have been found in virtually every canine breed; however, Poodles, Cocker Spaniels, Dachshunds, Beagles, and Boston Terriers may be predisposed.

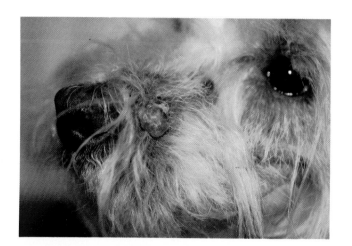

Figure 12-81   *Lobulated sebaceous adenoma on muzzle of 14-year-old male West Highland White Terrier.*

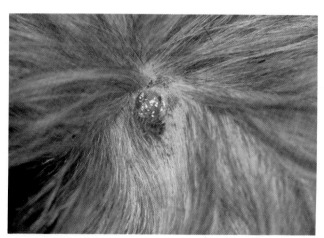

Figure 12-82   *Ulcerated sebaceous adenoma on head of 11-year-old male Skye Terrier.*

Sebaceous Adenocarcinoma

DESCRIPTION

1. Sebaceous adenocarcinomas are firm and poorly circumscribed
2. The tumor surface is usually alopecic and ulcerated
3. Tumor size ranges from 1 cm to greater than 6 cm in diameter

LOCATION

Sebaceous adenocarcinomas may occur anywhere on the body, but the head is the most common site.

BIOLOGIC BEHAVIOR

These tumors may recur at the site of surgical excision; however, metastasis to regional lymph nodes and the lungs is very rare.

COMMENTS

Sebaceous adenocarcinomas are common in the dog and very rare in the cat. The age of affected dogs varies, but most patients are 8 years of age or older. Cocker Spaniels may be at increased risk.

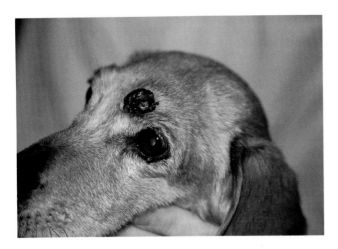

Figure 12-83 *Ulcerated sebaceous adenocarcinoma on head of 15-year-old female Dachshund.*

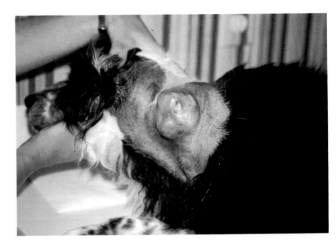

Figure 12-84 *Multinodular sebaceous adenocarcinoma with osseous metaplasia on neck of 12-year-old mixed-breed dog.*

Skin Tag (Fibrovascular Papilloma, Soft Fibroma)

DESCRIPTION

1. Skin tags vary greatly in their appearance
2. They are usually soft and pedunculated
3. They may be corrugated or smooth
4. Many are hyperpigmented
5. Skin tags may be solitary or multiple
6. Size ranges from less than 1 cm to several centimeters in length

LOCATION

Skin tags may occur anywhere on the body, but the ventral thorax and proximal extremities are sites of predilection.

BIOLOGIC BEHAVIOR

Skin tags are benign. They do not recur at the site of surgical excision and they do not metastasize.

COMMENTS

Skin tags are common canine tumors. No age or sex predisposition has been documented. They tend to occur in larger breeds of dogs.

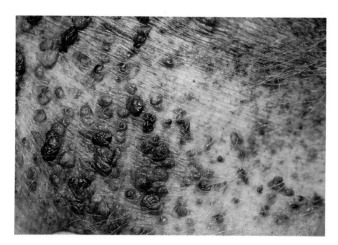

Figure 12-85 *Nonpigmented, 2.5 cm skin tag in axillary area of young Pit Bull Terrier.*

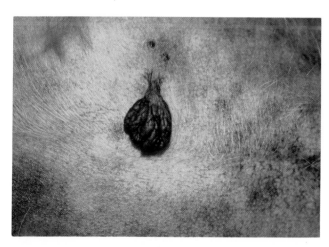

Figure 12-86 *Pigmented, pedunculated, lobulated skin tag on ventral thorax of 9-year-old Lhasa Apso. (Subcutaneous hemorrhage surrounding lesion was caused by injection of lidocaine.)*

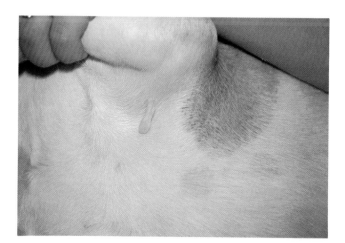

Figure 12-87 *Multiple, small, pigmented skin tags on flank of 11-year-old German Shepherd Dog.*

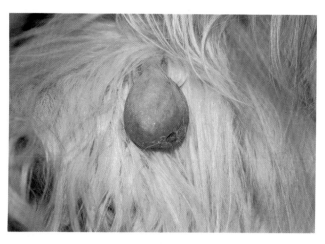

Figure 12-88 *Pedunculated, ulcerated skin tag on medial aspect of right foreleg of English Springer Spaniel.*

Squamous Cell Carcinoma

DESCRIPTION

1. Squamous cell carcinoma may appear as a papillary, proliferative growth usually with an ulcerated surface
2. The tumor may also appear as an erosive, ulcerative lesion
3. The tumor borders are usually poorly defined
4. Tumors are usually solitary
5. Size ranges from less than 1 cm to several centimeters in diameter

LOCATION

In dogs squamous cell carcinomas are most frequently found on the limbs; however, they may occur anywhere on the body. In cats the tumors are most common on the face and ears.

BIOLOGIC BEHAVIOR

These tumors are locally invasive. Metastasis to regional lymph nodes and the lungs may occur. Digital canine squamous cell carcinomas have been reported to have the greatest tendency to metastasize.

COMMENTS

Squamous cell carcinomas are common in the dog and cat. Older animals are predisposed. No sex predilection has been documented. White cats are reported to have greater than 10 times the incidence of squamous cell carcinoma when compared to cats of other colors. Predisposed canine breeds include Boxers, Poodles, Scottish Terriers, and Pekingese. Excessive exposure to ultraviolet light has been shown to produce these tumors in both dogs and cats.

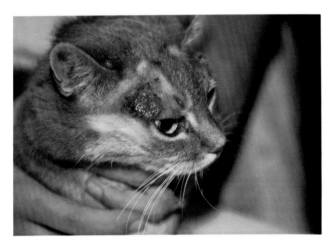

Figure 12-89 *Fifteen-year-old cat with ulcerative squamous cell carcinoma.*

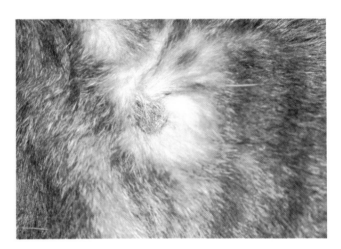

Figure 12-90 *Another squamous cell carcinoma on shoulder of patient shown in Figure 12-89.*

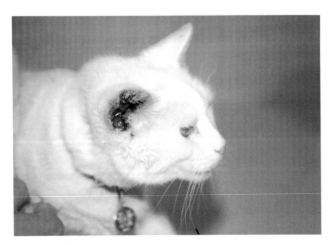

Figure 12-91 *Severely ulcerated necrotic ear pinna of 7-year-old cat. This patient's squamous cell carcinoma was believed to be caused by excessive exposure to sunlight.*

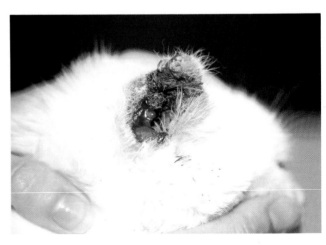

Figure 12-92 *Closer view of squamous cell carcinoma shown in Figure 12-91.*

Transmissible Venereal Tumor

DESCRIPTION

1. Most tumors are cauliflower like in appearance, but they may be nodular or pedunculated
2. They are usually quite friable and bleed easily
3. They may have an ulcerated and/or necrotic surface
4. Color ranges from off-white to red
5. Tumors may be solitary or multiple
6. Size ranges from 0.5 to 10 cm in diameter

LOCATION

Transmissible venereal tumors are most frequently located on the penis or in the vagina. The oral cavity and skin may also be involved.

BIOLOGIC BEHAVIOR

Transmissible venereal tumors grow rapidly, are locally invasive, and may metastasize to regional lymph nodes, the lungs, and viscera. Spontaneous remission of naturally occurring transmissible venereal tumors has not been documented.

COMMENTS

Transmissible venereal tumor is uncommon in the dog. It has not been reported in the cat. There are no age, breed, or sex predispositions. Young, sexually active canines are at significantly increased risk. Transmission occurs from one dog to another by coitus, licking, scratching, and biting.

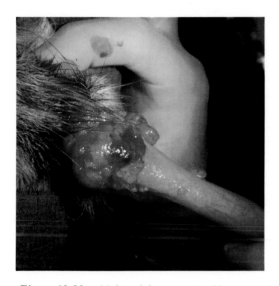

Figure 12-93   *Multinodular transmissible venereal tumor on penis of 3-year-old mixed-breed dog. (Slide courtesy of Dr. David Saylor, Gaithersburg, Maryland.)*

Trichoepithelioma

DESCRIPTION

1. Tumors vary in shape, but most are round to oval
2. They are usually firm and well circumscribed
3. Some tumors do not extend above the skin surface; others are nodular or pedunculated
4. The surface is usually ulcerated and alopecic
5. Tumors may be solitary or multiple.
6. Size ranges from less than 1 cm up to 10 cm in diameter

LOCATION

In dogs trichoepitheliomas occur most frequently on the back. In cats the head is the most common site of occurrence.

BIOLOGIC BEHAVIOR

Trichoepitheliomas are considered to be benign. Recurrence at the site of surgical excision and metastasis to local lymph nodes and lungs are rare.

COMMENTS

Trichoepitheliomas are uncommon in the dog and rare in the cat. No breed or sex predilection has been documented. Most tumors occur in patients over 5 years of age.

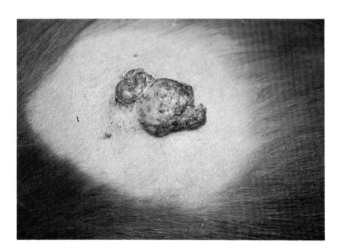

Figure 12-94 *Multinodular trichoepithelioma on back of 8-year-old female Golden Retriever.*

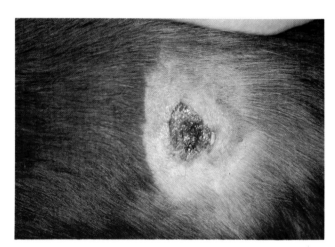

Figure 12-95 *Ulcerated, infected trichoepithelioma on rump of 4-year-old mixed-breed dog.*

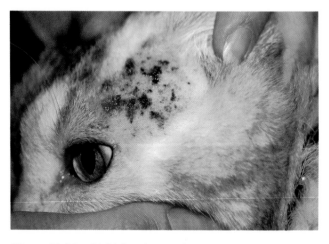

Figure 12-96 *Multiple, pigmented, invasive trichoepithelioma in preauricular area of 12-year-old cat.*

INDEX